Plant-Based Breakfast on a Budget

Cheap and Easy Plant-Based Breakfast Recipes to Save Your Money and Boost Your Day

Carl Brady

Table of contents

Tofu Scramble

Preparation time: 5 minutes Cooking time: 18 minutes
Servings: 4

Ingredients:

For The Spice Mix: 1 teaspoon black salt

1/4 teaspoon garlic powder

1 teaspoon red chili powder

1 teaspoon ground cumin

3/4 teaspoons turmeric

2 tablespoons nutritional yeast

For The Tofu Scramble:

2 cups cooked black beans

16 ounces tofu, firm, pressed, drained

1 chopped red pepper

1 1/2 cups sliced button mushrooms

1/2 of white onion, chopped

1 teaspoon minced garlic

1 tablespoon olive oil

Directions:

Take a skillet pan, place it over medium-high heat, add oil and when hot, add onion, pepper, mushrooms, and garlic and cook for 8 minutes until golden. Meanwhile, prepare the spice mix and for this, place all its ingredients in a bowl and stir until combined. When vegetables have cooked, add tofu in it, crumble it, then add black beans, sprinkle with prepared spice mix, stir and cook for 8 minutes until hot. Serve straight away.

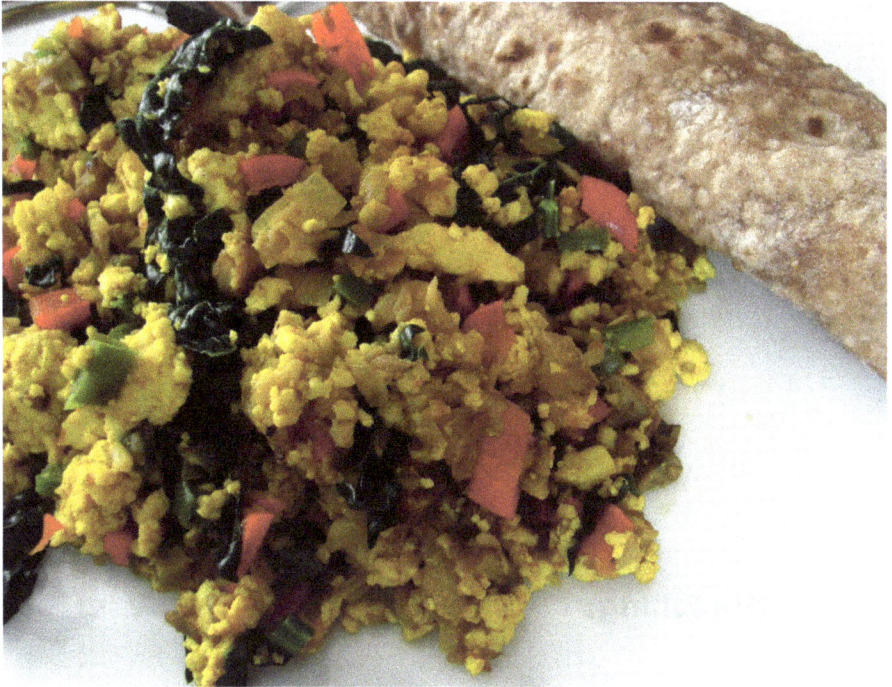

Tomato and Asparagus Quiche

Preparation time: 40 minutes Cooking time: 35 minutes

Servings: 12

Ingredients:

For the Dough:

2 cups whole wheat flour

1/2 teaspoon salt

3/4 cup vegan margarine

1/3 cup water

For the Filling:

14 oz silken tofu

6 cherry tomatoes, halved

2 green onions, cut into rings

10 sun-dried tomatoes, in oil, chopped

7 oz green asparagus, diced

1 1/2 tablespoons herbs de Provence

1 tablespoon cornstarch

1 teaspoon turmeric

3 tablespoons olive oil

Directions:

Switch on the oven, then set it to 350 degrees F and let it preheat. Pre the dough and for this, take a bowl, place all the ingredients for it, beat until incorporated, then knead for 5 minutes until smooth and refrigerate the dough for 30 minutes. Meanwhile, take a skillet pan, place it over medium heat, add 1 tablespoon oil and when hot, add green onion and cook for 2 minutes, set aside until required. Place a pot half full wit salty water over medium heat, bring it to boil, then add asparagus and boil for 3 minutes until tender, drain and set aside until required. Take a medium bowl, add tofu along with herbs de Provence, starch, turmeric, and oil, whisk until smooth and then fold in tomatoes, green onion, and asparagus until mixed. Divide the prepared dough into twelve sections, take a muffin tray, line it twelve cups with baking cups, and then press a dough ball at the bottom of each cup and all the way up. Fill the cups with prepared tofu mixture, top with tomatoes, and bake for 35 minutes until cooked. Serve straight away.

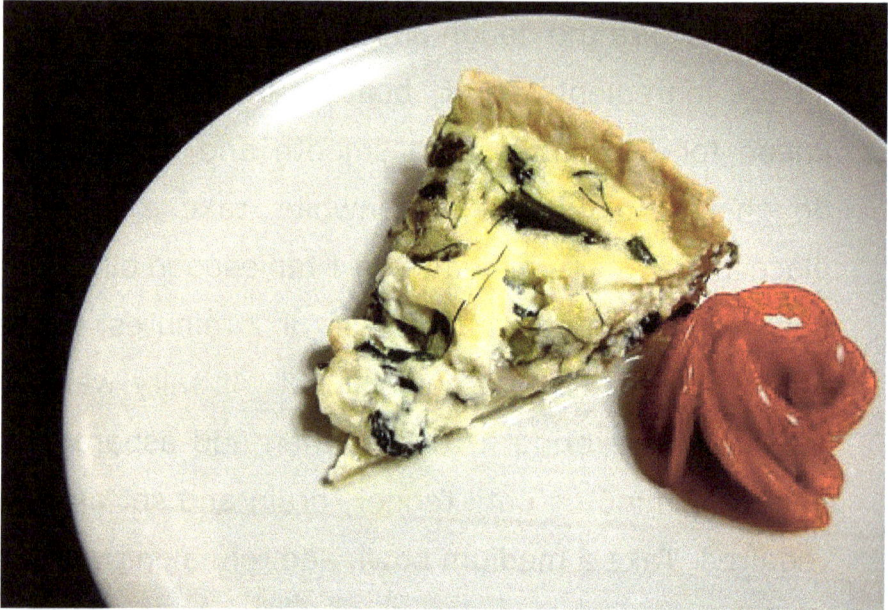

Chickpeas On Toast

Preparation time: 5 minutes Cooking time: 15 minutes Servings: 6

Ingredients:

14-oz cooked chickpeas

1 cup baby spinach

1/2 cup chopped white onion

1 cup crushed tomatoes

½ teaspoon minced garlic

¼ teaspoon ground black pepper

1/2 teaspoon brown sugar

1 teaspoon smoked paprika powder

1/3 teaspoon sea salt

1 tablespoon olive oil

6 slices of gluten-free bread, toasted

Directions:

Take a frying pan, place it over medium heat, add oil and when hot, add onion and cook for 2 minutes. Then stir in garlic, cook for 30 seconds until fragrant, stir in paprika and continue cooking for 10 seconds. Add tomatoes, stir, bring the mixture to simmer, season with black pepper, sugar, and salt and then stir in chickpeas. Sir, in spinach, cook for 2 minutes until leaves have wilted, then remove the pan from heat and taste to adjust seasoning. Serve cooked chickpeas on toasted bread.

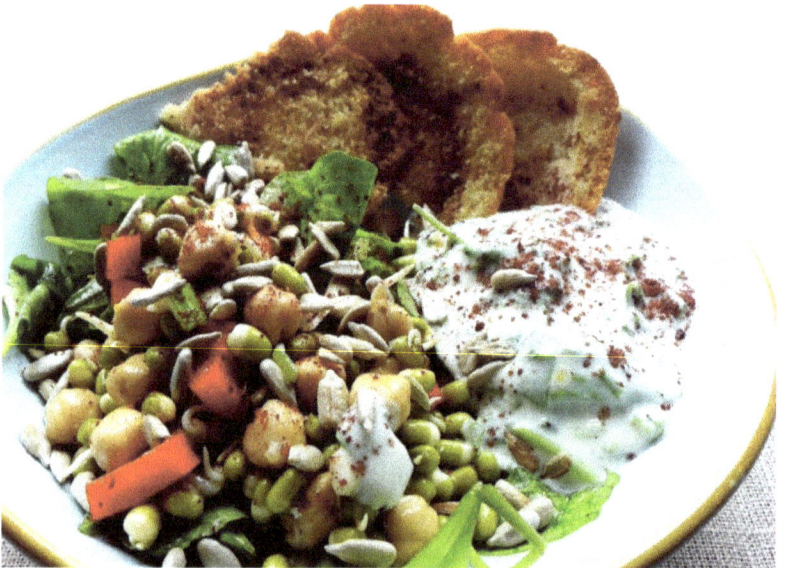

Ultimate Breakfast Sandwich

Preparation time: 40 minutes Cooking time: 10 minutes Servings: 4

Ingredients:

For the Tofu:

12 ounces tofu, extra-firm, pressed, drain

1/2 teaspoon garlic powder

1 teaspoon liquid smoke

2 tablespoons nutritional yeast

1 teaspoon Sriracha sauce

2 tablespoons soy sauce

2 tablespoons olive oil

2 tablespoons water

For the Vegan Breakfast Sandwich:

1 large tomato, sliced

4 English muffins, halved, toasted

1 avocado, mashed

Directions: Prepare tofu, and for this, cut tofu into four slices and set aside. Stir together remaining ingredients of tofu, pour the mixture into a bag, then add tofu pieces, toss until coated and marinate for 30 minutes. Take a skillet pan, place it over medium-high heat, add tofu slices along with the marinade and cook for 5 minutes per side. Prepare sandwich and for this, spread mashed avocado on the inner of the muffin, top with a slice of tofu, layer with a tomato slice and then serve.

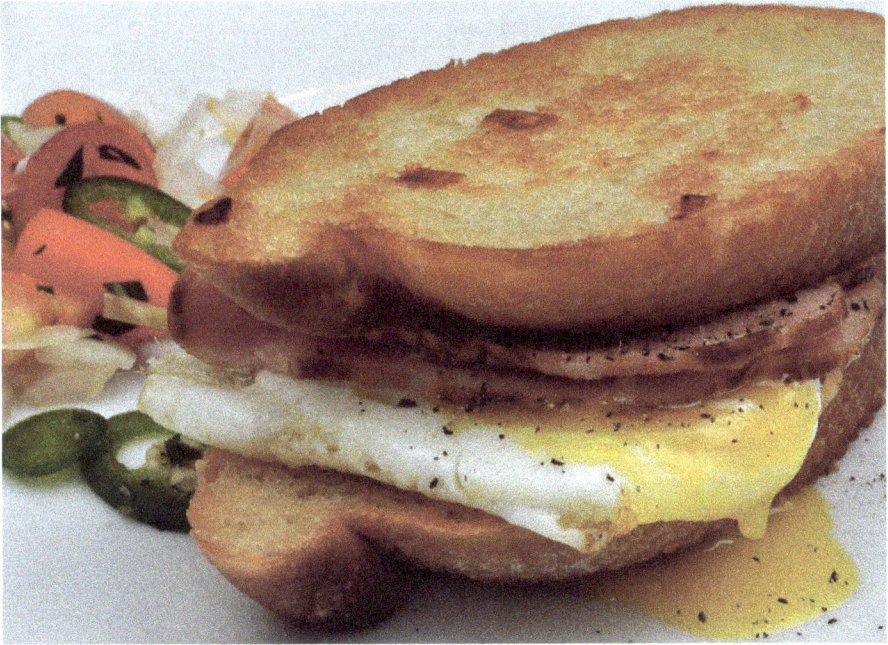

Chickpea Omelet

Preparation time: 5 minutes Cooking time: 10 minutes
Servings: 1

Ingredients:

3 Tablespoon chickpea flour

1 small white onion, peeled, diced

½ teaspoon black salt

2 tablespoons chopped the dill

2 tablespoons chopped basil

1/8 teaspoon ground black pepper

2 Tablespoon olive oil 8 Tablespoon water

Directions:

Take a bowl, add flour in it along with salt and black
pepper, stir until mixed, and then whisk in water until
creamy. Take a skillet pan, place it over medium heat,
add 1 tablespoon oil and when hot, add onion and cook
for 4 minutes until cooked. Add onion to omelet mixture

and then stir until combined. Add remaining oil into the pan, pour in prepared batter, spread evenly, and cook for 3 minutes per side until cooked. Serve omelet with bread.

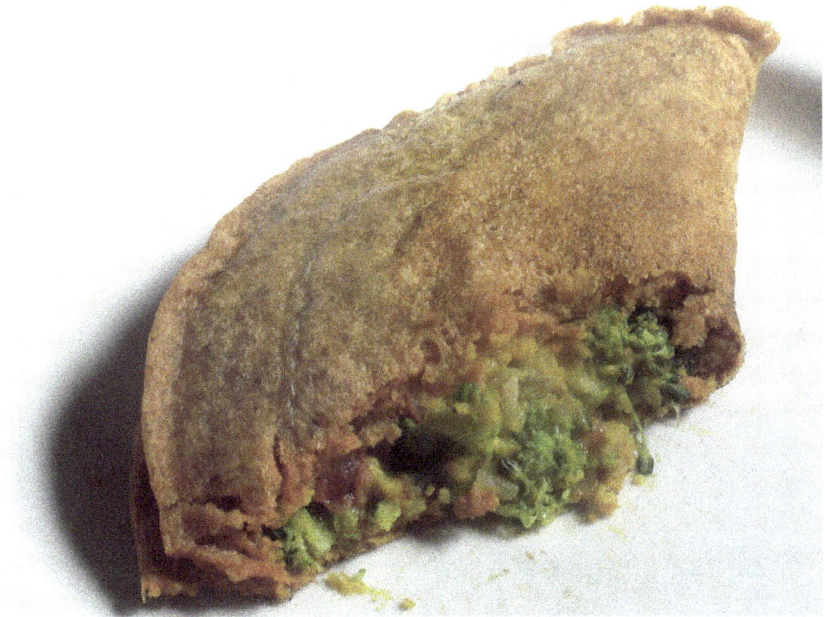

Pancake

Preparation time: 10 minutes Cooking time: 18 minutes

Servings: 4

Ingredients:

Dry Ingredients:

1 cup buckwheat flour

1/8 teaspoon salt

½ teaspoon gluten-free baking powder

½ teaspoon baking soda

Wet Ingredients:

1 tablespoon almond butter

2 tablespoon maple syrup

1 tablespoon lime juice

1 cup coconut milk, unsweetened

Directions: Take a medium bowl, add all the dry ingredients and stir until mixed. Take another bowl, place all the wet ingredients, whisk until combined, and then gradually whisk in dry ingredients mixture until smooth and incorporated. Take a frying pan, place it over medium heat, add 2 teaspoons oil and when hot, drop in batter and cook for 3 minutes per side until cooked and lightly browned. Serve pancakes and fruits and maple syrup.

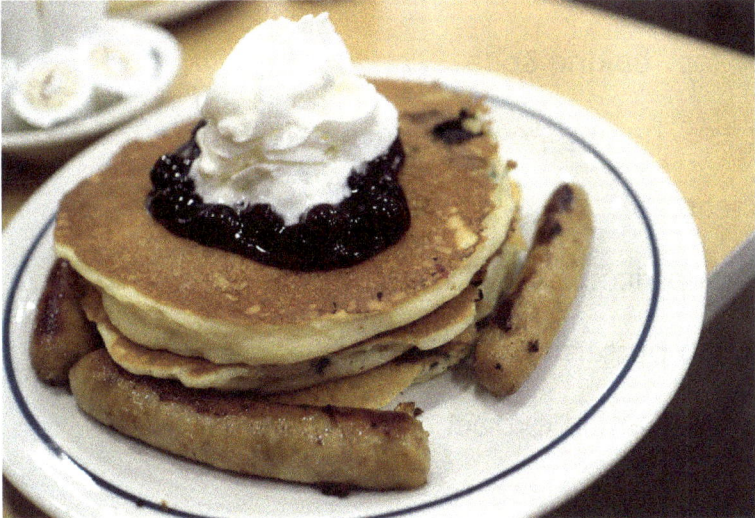

Apple Pancakes

Preparation Time: 15 minutes Cooking Time: 4 minutes

Servings: 4

Ingredients:

1 cup whole-wheat flour

¾ tsp. ground cinnamon, divided

¼ tsp. baking soda

1 tsp. baking powder Pinch salt

1 egg

¾ cup ricotta cheese

1 cup buttermilk

1 tsp. vanilla extract

1 tbsp. sugar and

1 tsp. sugar, divided

1 apple, sliced into rings

4 tsp. butter

4 tsp. walnut oil

Directions: In a bowl, mix the flour, ½ teaspoon cinnamon, baking soda, baking powder and salt. In another bowl, beat the eggs and stir in the cheese, milk, vanilla and 1 tablespoon sugar. Gradually add the second bowl to the first one. Mix well. Combine the remaining cinnamon and 1 teaspoon sugar in a separate dish. Coat each apple ring with this mixture. Pour the butter and oil in a pan over medium heat. Add the apples and pour the batter around the apple. Cook for 2 minutes. Flip and cook for another 2 minutes.

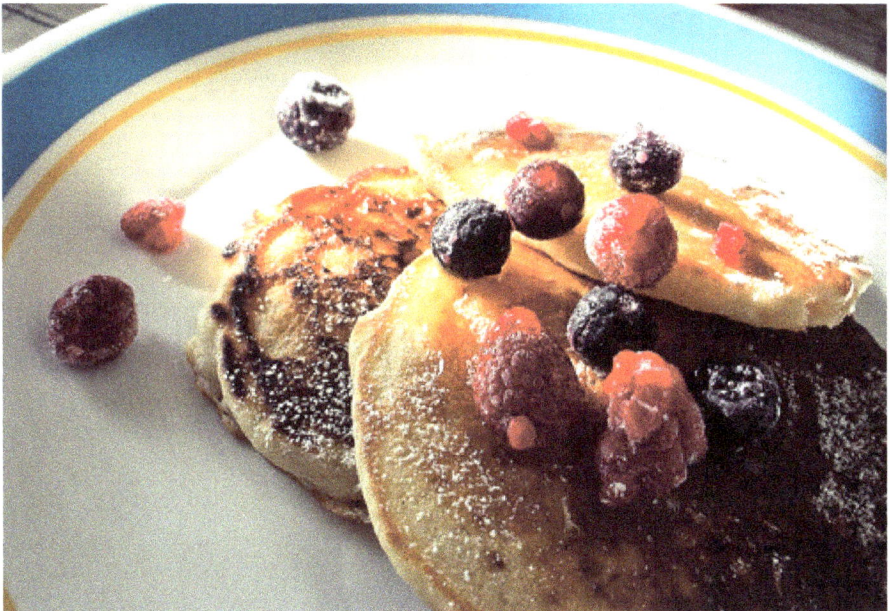

Herb & Cheese Omelet

Preparation Time: 5 minutes Cooking Time: 5 minutes

Servings: 2

Ingredients:

4 eggs Salt and pepper to taste

2 tbsp. low-fat milk

1 tsp. chives, chopped

1 tbsp. parsley, chopped

½ cup goat cheese, crumbled

1 tsp. olive oil

Directions:

Beat the eggs in a bowl. Stir in the salt, pepper and milk. In a bowl, combine the chives, parsley and goat cheese. Pour the oil into a pan over medium heat. Cook the eggs for 3 minutes. Add the cheese mixture on top. Fold and serve.

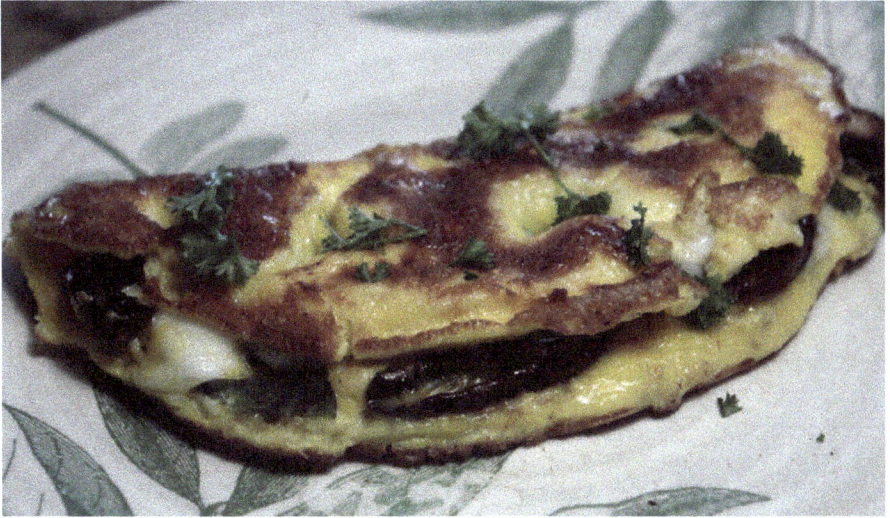

Quinoa Sensation Early Morning Porridge

Preparation time: 5 minutes Cooking time: 10 minutes

Servings: 3

Ingredients:

½ cup quinoa

3 tbsp. brown sugar

½ tsp. cinnamon

2 cups almond milk

½ cup water dash of salt

Directions:

Begin by heating the quinoa in a saucepan over medium heat. Add the cinnamon, and cook the quinoa until it's sufficiently toasted. This should take about five minutes. Afterwards, add the remaining ingredients. Bring the mixture to a boil. Next, place the stovetop to low heat, and allow the mixture to simmer for thirty minutes. If you need to, you can add more water if the porridge dries too quickly. Make sure to stir every few seconds. Enjoy!

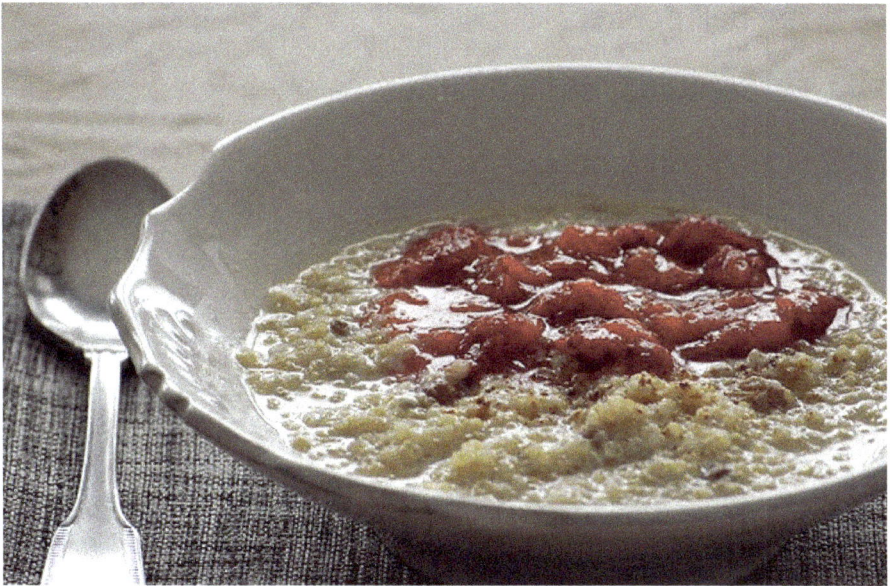

Green Breakfast Salad

Preparation Time: 10 minutes Cooking time: 10 minutes
Servings: 4

Ingredients:

1 tablespoon lemon juice

4 red bell peppers

1 lettuce head, cut into strips

Salt and black pepper to the taste

3 tablespoons coconut cream

2 tablespoons olive oil

1 ounces rocket leaves

Directions:

Place bell pepper in your air fryer's basket, cook at 400 degrees F for 10 minutes, transfer to a bowl, leave them aside to cool down, peel, cut them in strips and put them in a bowl. Add rocket leaves and lettuce strips and toss. In a bowl, mix oil with lemon juice, coconut cream, salt and pepper, whisk well, add over the salad, toss to coat, divide between plates and serve for breakfast. Enjoy!

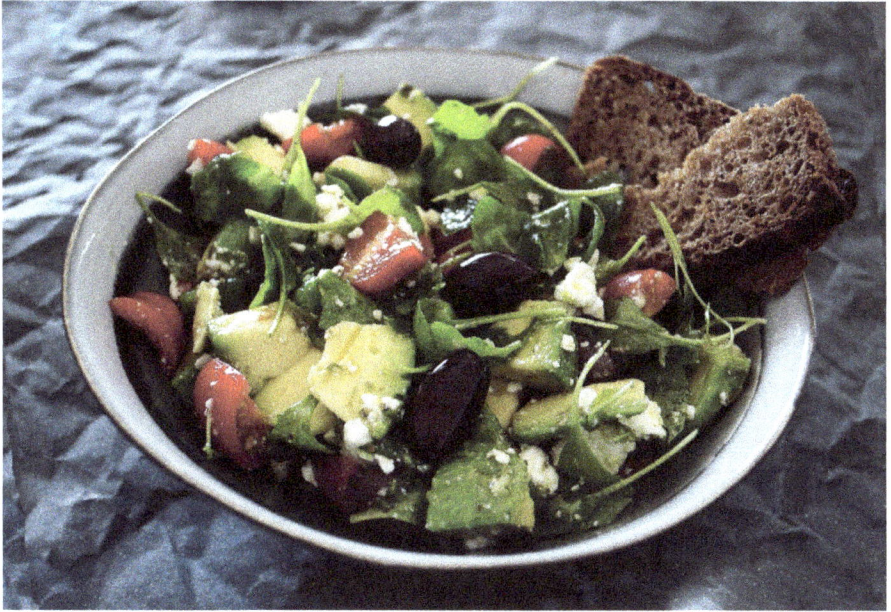

Pita Bread

Servings: 8 pitas Preparation Time: 15 mins Cooking Time: 6 mins

Ingredients:

2 cups whole wheat flour

1 cup all-purpose flour

2½ teaspoons quick-acting yeast

1½ cups + 2 tablespoons lukewarm water

1 tablespoon olive oil

Directions:

Add all the dry Ingredients into a large bowl. Keep the east as far as possible from the salt.

Add in the olive oil and enough of the water to make a firm, smooth dough. You might not need all of the water or you might need more, it depends on the humidity levels and brand of flour.

Stir well until the all the flour is absorbed, to form a shaggy dough.

Scrape the dough onto a clean, dry surface. Oil the work surface and hands with some olive oil. This will make the dough easier to handle while kneading. Knead for 7 - 10 minutes, until the dough becomes smoother and less sticky.

Keep going until the dough slowly but easily bounces back to shape when poked. Divide the dough into 8 portions. Roll each piece about 3mm thick. Place on a lightly floured baking sheet and cover with clean, dry-damp kitchen towels.

Rest for 30 minutes. Preheat the oven to 500 degrees Fahrenheit and after 30 minutes uncover the pitas and gently flip over. You will need to peel the breads off the baking tray but they'll come up easily as the tray is floured. Bake for 5 - 6 minutes until they are puffed but not at all colored.

Cover with a kitchen towel and leave to coo. These pita breads will soften as they cool.

Recipe Notes: These Pita Breads keep well for 2 - 3 days but can also be frozen. Place in a Ziploc bag and seal. To reheat pop straight in the oven from frozen at 350 degrees Fahrenheit for about 5 minutes.

The salt in this recipe is optional.

Omitting it will affect the flavor slightly, but not the recipe.

The oil is also optional.

If you omit it, add an extra tablespoon of water to compensate.

If you do not add oil to the recipe the pita bread won't be as soft and will stale slightly quicker as oil is a preservative.

Without oil, its best to freeze the breads and then reheat them when you need them.

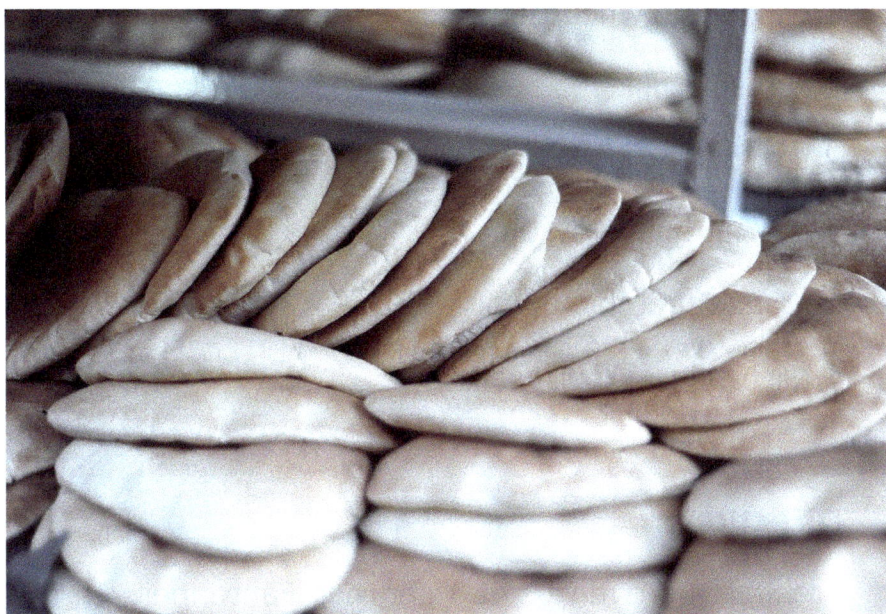

Wheat Quick Bread

Servings: 1 loaf Preparation Time: 10 mins Cooking Time: 20 mins

Ingredients:

1 cup rolled oats

1 cup whole wheat flour

1 cup soy milk

2 tsp. baking powder

1½ tbsp. agave syrup

1 tbsp. vegetable oil

1 tsp. salt

Directions:

Preheat the oven to 450 degrees Fahrenheit. In a food processor or blender, grind the oatmeal to make oatmeal flour. Combine oatmeal flour, whole wheat flour, baking powder and salt. In a separate bowl, dissolve the agave syrup in vegetable oil, and then stir in the soy milk. Combine both the dry and wet mixtures and stir until they form a soft dough. Form the dough into a smooth round ball and place on a lightly oiled baking sheet. Bake in for 20 minutes, or until the bottom crust of loaf sounds hollow when tapped.

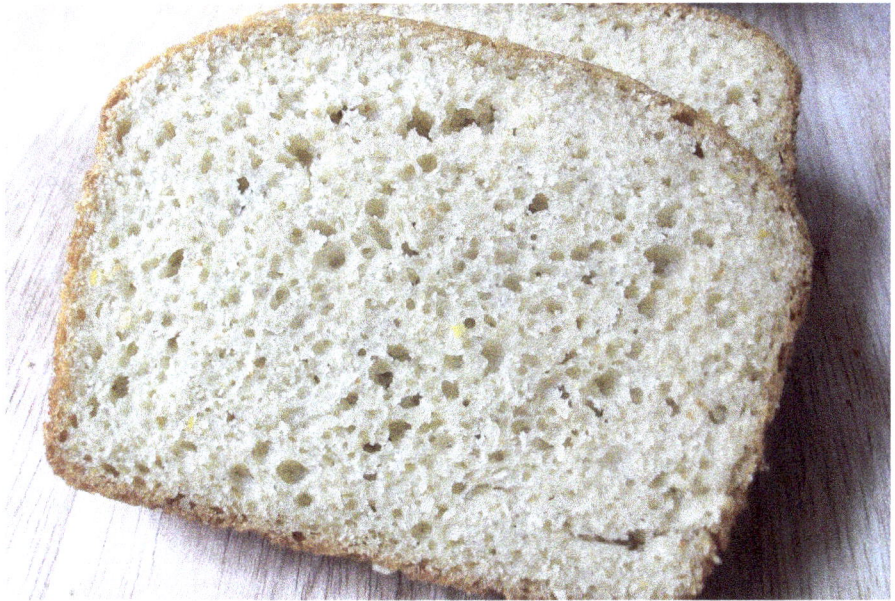

Carrotastic Apple Muffins

Preparation time: 5 minutes Cooking time: 40 minutes Servings: 12.

Ingredients:

2 ¾ cups all-purpose flour

4 tsp. baking soda

1 cup brown sugar

1/3 cup white sugar

4 tsp. cinnamon

2 tsp. salt

1 tsp. baking powder

2 ½ cups grated carrots

2 cored, peeled, and shredded apples

1 1/3 cups applesauce

1/3 cup vegetable oil

6 tsp. dry egg replacer

Directions:

Begin by preheating your oven to 375 degrees Fahrenheit. Next, mix together the two sugars, the baking soda, the baking powder, the flour, the cinnamon, and the salt. Stir well. To the side, mix together the applesauce, the egg substitute, and the oil. Stir well, and add the dry ingredients to the wet ingredients. Spoon this created mixture into muffin tins, and bake the muffins for twenty minutes. Allow them to cool prior to serving, and enjoy!

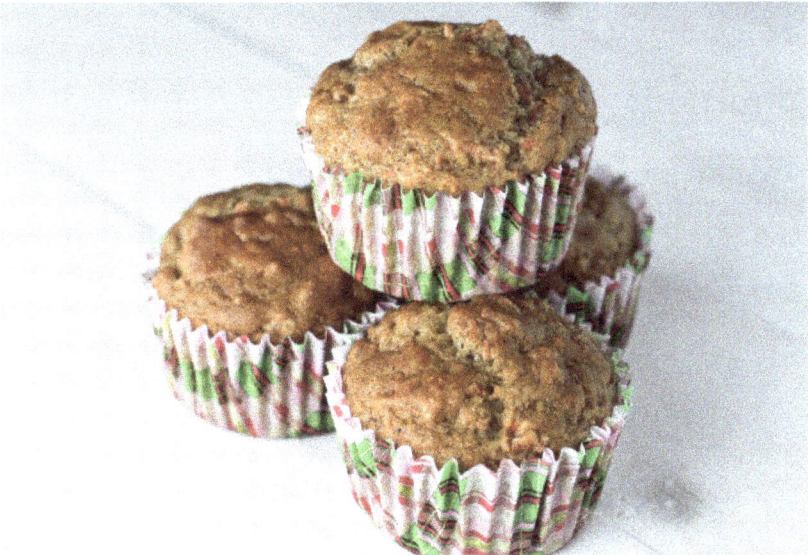

Sweet Pomegranate Porridge

Preparation time: 5 minutes Cooking time: 30 minutes

Servings: 4

Ingredients:

2 Cups Oats

1 ½ Cups Water

1 ½ Cups Pomegranate Juice

2 Tablespoons Pomegranate Molasses

Directions:

Pour all ingredients into the instant pot and mix well. Seal the lid, and cook on high pressure for four minutes. Use a quick release, and serve warm.

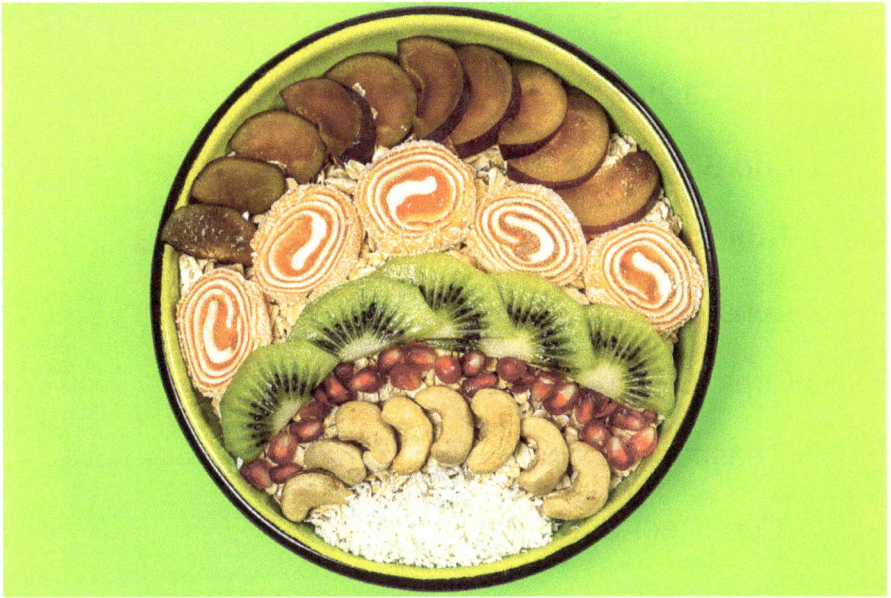

Apple Oatmeal

Preparation time: 5 minutes Cooking time: 20 minutes

Servings: 4

Ingredients:

¼ Teaspoon Sea Salt

1 Cup Cashew Milk

1 Cup Strawberries, Halved & Fresh

1 Tablespoon Brown Sugar

2 Cups Apples, Diced

3 Cups Water

¼ Teaspoon Coconut Oil

½ Cup Steel Cut Oats

Directions:

Start by greasing your instant pot with oil, and add everything to it except for the milk and berries. Lock the lid and cook on high pressure for ten minutes. Allow for a natural pressure release, and then add in your milk and strawberries. Mix well, and serve warm.

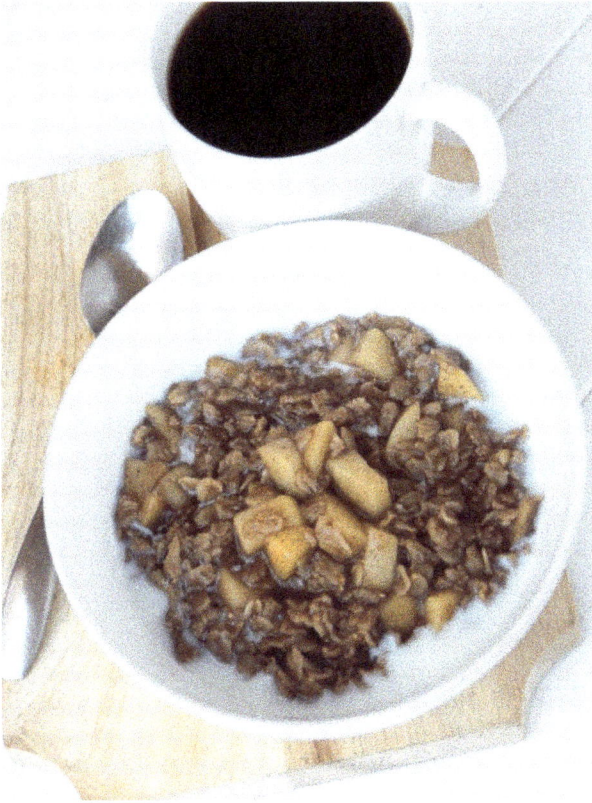

Potato and Zucchini Omelet

Preparation time: 5 minutes Cooking time: 20 minutes

Ingredients:

½ lb. potato (about 1¼ cups diced)

½ lb. zucchini (about 1½ cups diced)

⅔ cup chopped onion (1 small)

1 Tbs. butter

2 Tbs. olive oil

¼ tsp. dried dill weed

¼ tsp. dried basil, crushed

½ tsp. crushed dried red

pepper salt to taste

fresh-ground black pepper to taste

5 to 6 eggs butter for frying garnish sour cream

Directions:

Peel or scrub the potato and cut it in ½-inch dice. Wash, trim, and finely dice the zucchini. Drop the diced potato into boiling salted water and cook for 5 minutes, then drain it and set it aside. Cook the diced zucchini in boiling water for 3 to 4 minutes, drain, and set aside. Heat the butter and the olive oil in a medium-sized skillet and sauté the onions in it until they start to color. Add the partially cooked potato and zucchini, the dill weed, basil, crushed red pepper, and salt. Cook this mixture over medium heat, stirring often, until the potatoes are just tender. Grind in some black pepper and add more salt if needed. Make either 2 medium-sized or 3 small omelets according to the directions. When the eggs are almost set, spoon some of the hot vegetables onto one side and fold the other side of the omelet over the filling. Slide the omelets out onto warm plates and serve immediately with sour cream.

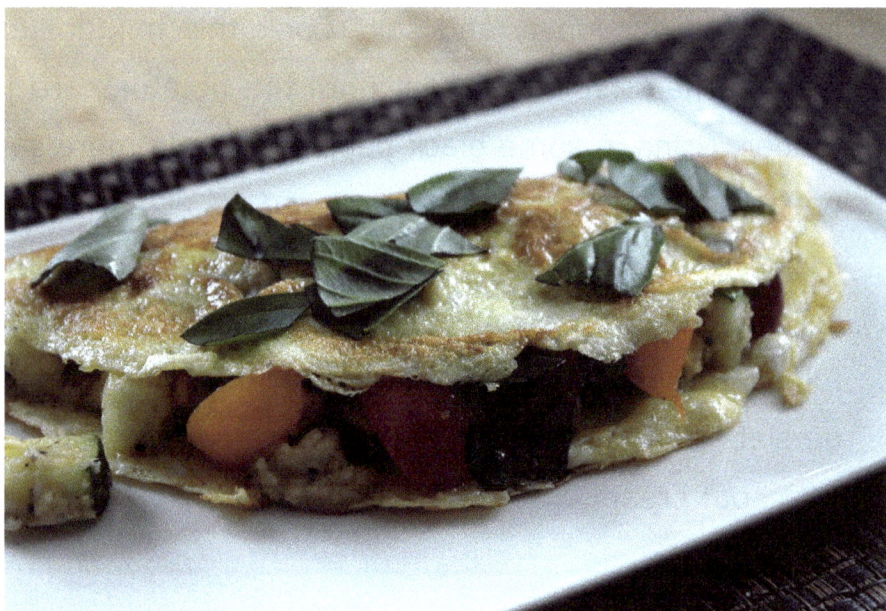

Creamy Roasted Plums

Preparation time: 5 minutes Cooking time: 30 minutes
Servings: 3

Ingredients:

1 teaspoon olive oil

4 ripe plums, halved and pitted

4 teaspoons sugar

1 cup vanilla yogurt

2 tablespoons fresh basil, finely chopped

1 teaspoon honey

Directions:

Preheat the oven to 400°F. Oil a large baking dish. Place the plums inside, cut side up, and sprinkle ½ teaspoon sugar over each. Bake, uncovered, for 35 minutes. While the plums are baking, stir together the yogurt, basil, and honey. Divide half of yogurt mixture onto each of 4 plates, or a large serving platter. When plums are finished baking, remove them from the oven and place 2 halves over yogurt on each plate. Fill the holes with remaining yogurt mixture and serve warm.

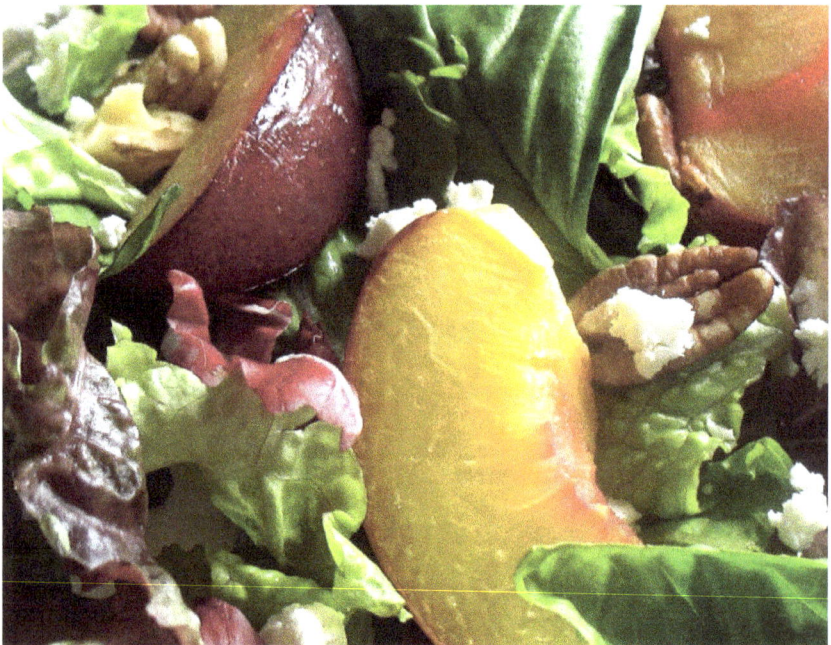

Tomato Omelet

Preparation time: 5 minutes Cooking time: 40 minutes
Servings: 3

Ingredients:

8 medium sized tomatoes

2 cloves garlic

2 bay leaves

½ tsp. dried tarragon, crushed

1 tsp. salt, and more to taste

2 Tbs. chopped fresh parsley

1 medium-sized yellow onion

3 Tbs. olive oil

½ tsp. dried basil, crushed

5 cured black olives, pitted and sliced

coarse ground black pepper to taste

8 to 10 eggs milk

Directions:

Blanch the tomatoes in boiling water for about 2 minutes and then peel them. Chop the tomatoes very coarsely and put them aside in a bowl with the salt. Chop the onion, mince the garlic, and sauté them in the olive oil in a large skillet until they begin to show color. Add the bay leaves and sauté a few minutes more. Add the tomatoes, the basil, tarragon, parsley, and sliced olives, and cook over medium heat, stirring occasionally, until the sauce is thick. It should take about 40 to 45 minutes. Make individual omelets according to the directions. Spoon on some of the hot Provençale sauce just when the eggs are nearly set. Blanch the tomatoes in boiling water for about 2 minutes and then peel them. Chop the tomatoes very coarsely and put them aside in a bowl with the salt. Chop the onion, mince the garlic, and sauté them in the olive oil in a large skillet until they begin to show color. Add the bay leaves and sauté a few minutes more. Add the tomatoes, the basil, tarragon, parsley, and sliced olives, and cook over medium heat, stirring occasionally, until the sauce is thick. It should take about 40 to 45 minutes. Make individual omelets according to the directions. Spoon on some of the hot Provençale sauce just when the eggs are nearly set, and fold the omelets over the sauce. Serve.

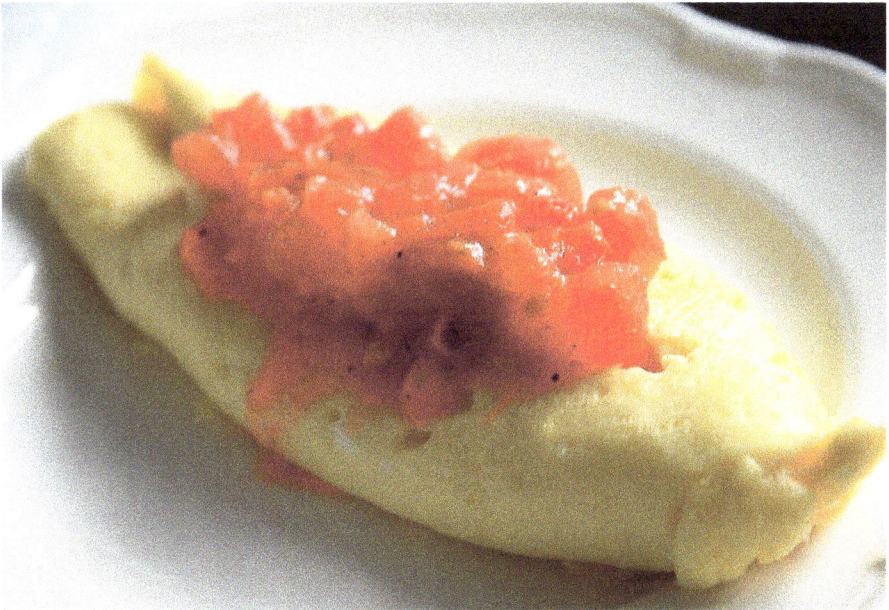

Italian Frittata

Preparation time: 5 minutes Cooking time: 40 minutes

Servings: 3

Ingredients:

6 large eggs, beaten

¼ cup extra-virgin olive oil

1 cup shitake mushrooms, cut very thin

½ medium yellow onion, cut very thin slices

1 large leeks, white and light green parts rinsed, chopped finely 8 basil leaves, torn

¼ cup Pecorino Romano, grated

1 teaspoon Unrefined Sea salt

Directions:

Preheat the oven to 350°F. Heat the oil in a large, wide, ovenproof skillet over medium-high heat. Add the onion and sauté, stirring occasionally, until softened and golden, 4 minutes. Add mushrooms and brown them, 4 minutes. Add the leeks, stir, and cook for another 4 minutes. Add the basil leaves, beaten eggs, Pecorino Romano, and salt. Mix well and reduce heat to medium-low. Cook, undisturbed, for 4 to 5 minutes, or until the eggs are cooked through. Finish off the frittata by putting the skillet in the oven until the frittata top is golden and the eggs are set. Cut into 4 and serve.

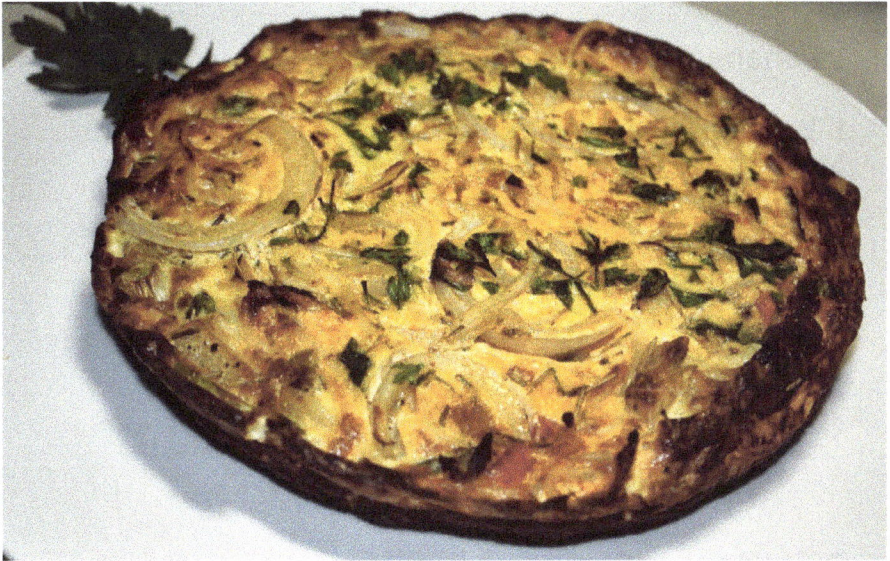

Vegan Tropical Pina Colada Smoothie

Preparation time: 5 minutes Cooking time: 0 minutes 1 smoothie.

Ingredients:

¾ cup soymilk

½ cup coconut milk

1 banana

1 ½ tbsp.. ground flax seed

1 tsp. vanilla

1 cup pineapple

1 tbsp. agave nectar

3 ice cubes

Directions:

Bring all the above ingredients together in a blender, and blend the ingredients to achieve your desired smoothie consistency. Enjoy!

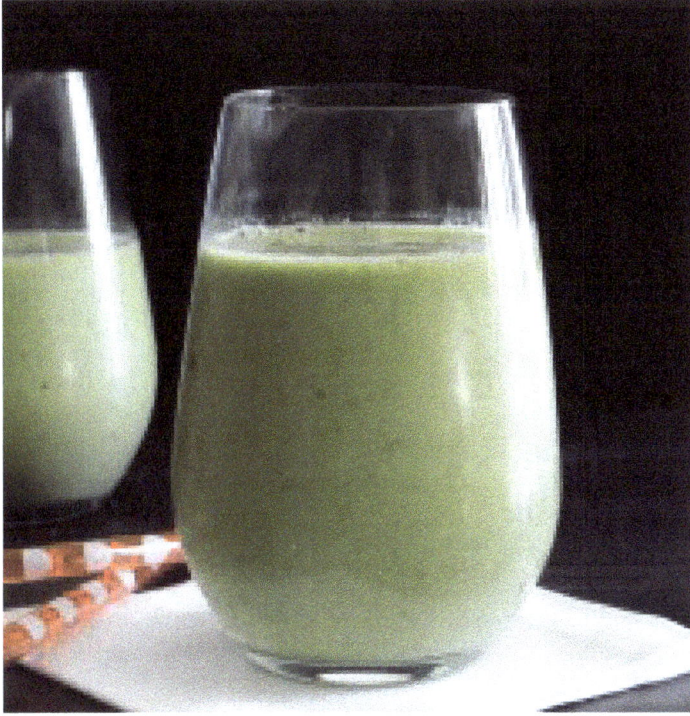

Mango Chia Smoothie

Preparation time: 5 minutes Cooking time: 0 minutes 1 Smoothie.

Ingredients:

1 peeled and chopped mango

1 sliced banana

1 tsp. flax seeds

½ tbsp. chia seeds

1 cup water

½ cup romaine lettuce

3 ice cubes

Directions:

Begin by bringing all the above ingredients together in a blender and blending them until they've reached your desired smoothie consistency. Enjoy!

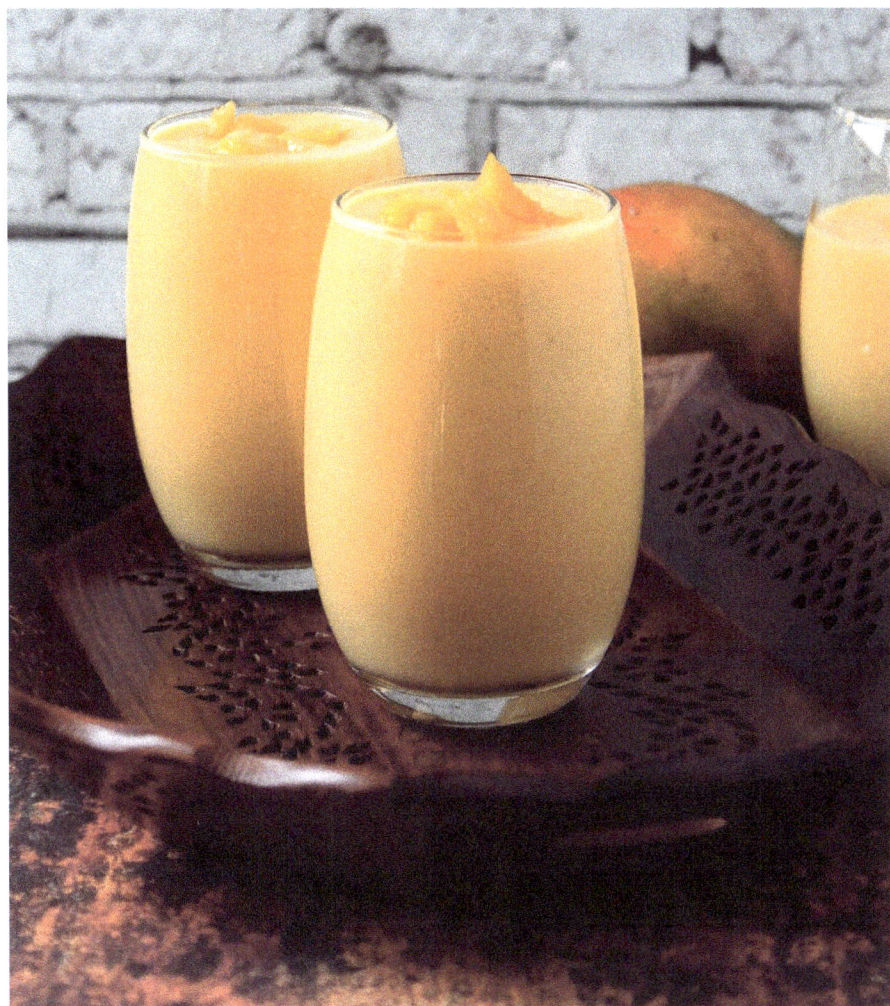

Peach Protein Bars

Servings: 6 Preparation Time: 60 min

Ingredients:

1 cup flax seeds

½ cup peanuts

¼ cup hemp seeds

15g dehydrated peaches

2 tbsp. psyllium husk

¼ tsp. stevia ½ tsp. salt

1¼ cup water

Directions:

Preheat oven at 350°F. Grind up nuts and seeds with ½ cup water in a blender, but make sure the mixture is not finely ground. Transfer and combine mixture with psyllium husk and cinnamon in a mixing bowl. Crush the dehydrated peaches into small bits and add to mixing bowl. Stir in the remaining water and salt until all Ingredients are combined. Let the mixture sit for a few minutes. Spread the mixture out on a baking sheet lined with parchment paper, and make sure the dough is about ¼ inch thick. Bake for 45 minutes, remove around 30 minutes to cut the dough carefully in six pieces, and bake for another 15 minutes. Remove from oven and cool for 30 minutes. Can be stored for a week or frozen up to two months.

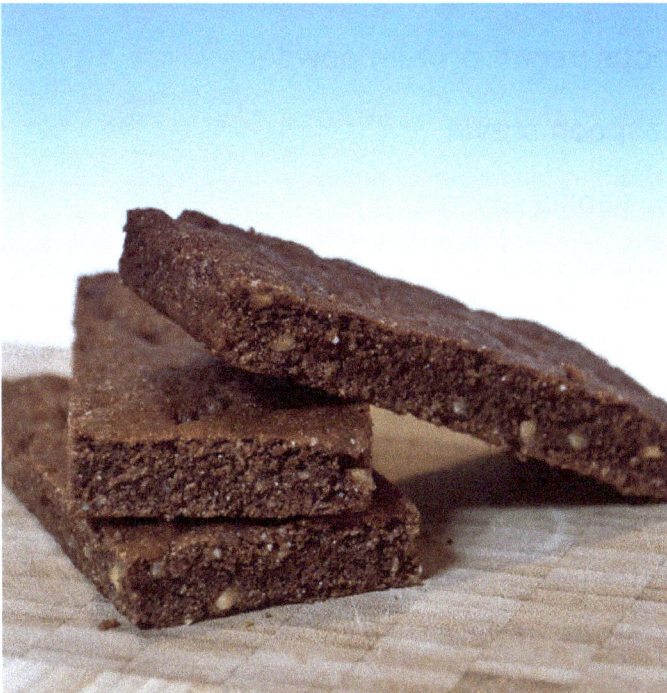

Breakfast Protein Bars

Servings: 16 Preparation Time: 35 min

Ingredients:

1 cup cashew cheese spread

2 tbsp. softened cocoa butter

4 tbsp. coconut flour

½ cup full fat coconut milk

2 scoops vegan protein powder

¼ teaspoon stevia

1 tsp. vanilla extract

Directions: Preheat oven to 375°F. Whisk together cocoa butter, cashew cheese spread, stevia, and coconut milk until mixed well. Stir the coconut flour and protein powder through until completely combined. Pour into a baking sheet lined with parchment paper, and bake for 30 minutes until the batter has set. Let it cool, and slice into 16 bars. Can be stored chilled for a week or frozen up to 2 months.

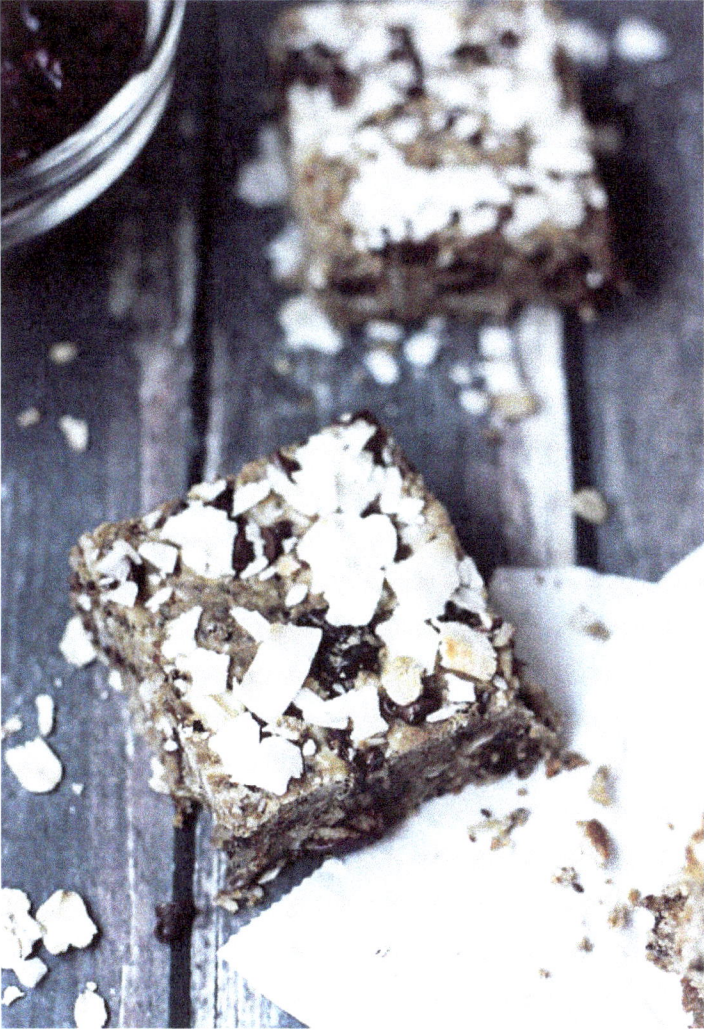

Breakfast Tacos

Preparation Time: 10 minutes Cooking time: 6 minutes

Servings: 4

Ingredients

½ cup grape tomatoes, quartered

1 avocado, sliced

8 corn tortillas Freshly ground black pepper

¼ teaspoon salt

¼ teaspoon cumin

¼ teaspoon ground turmeric

1 package firm tofu

1 garlic clove, minced

1 red pepper, diced

1 teaspoon olive oil

Directions: Heat oil in a skillet over medium heat. Add in garlic and red pepper and sauté for around 2 minutes. Using your hands, crumble the tofu and add into the pan;

and then add the seasonings. Cook for around 5 minutes making sure that you stir frequently. Taste and adjust the seasonings then apportion it and store in containers for the week. When you want to serve, simply put the scramble on tortillas, add any other toppings and enjoy.

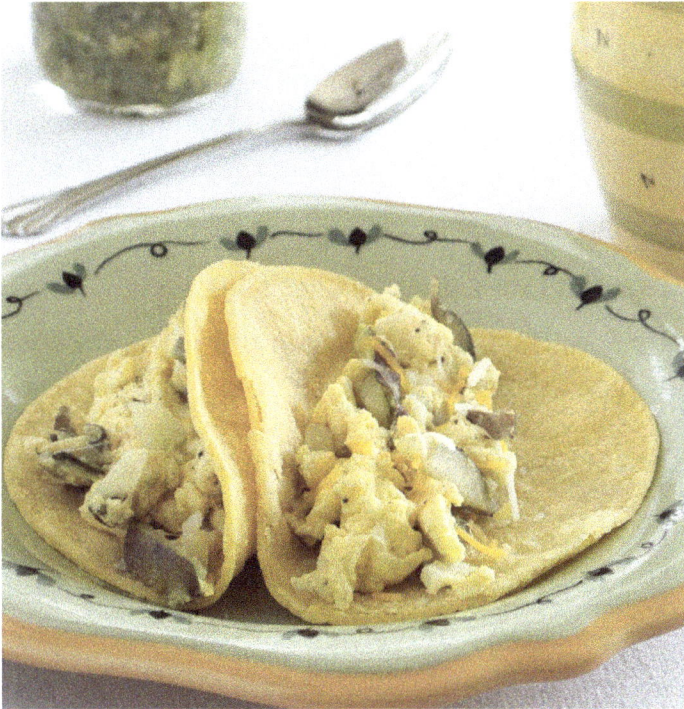

Poached Eggs

Preparation time: 5 minutes Cooking time: 30 minutes
Servings: 3

Ingredients:

1 large egg

1 teaspoon kosher salt

2 teaspoons of white vinegar

Directions: Place water in a deep 2-quart saucier until the water level is at an inch up the sides. Add salt and white vinegar. Set heat to medium and bring water to a simmer. Crack one large fresh egg into a custard cup and then use a spoon or a spatula handle to stir water in one direction until you see i's smoothly spinning around like a whirlpool. Carefully drop the egg right into the center of the swirl. The movement of the water will keep the egg whites from spreading out. Turn off heat. Cover pan and then set timer for exactly 5 minutes. Do not disturb the pan in any way. Remove egg using a slotted spoon. Immediately serve.

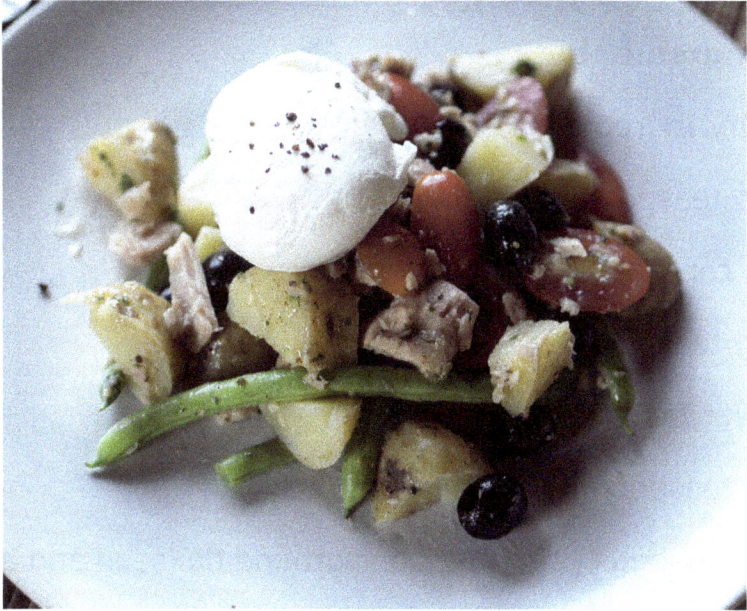

Breakfast Cookies

Preparation Time: 10 minutes Cooking time: 6 minutes

Makes 24-32

Ingredients

Dry Ingredients

½ teaspoon baking powder

2 cups rolled oats

½ teaspoon baking soda

Wet Ingredients

1 teaspoon pure vanilla extract

2 flax eggs (2 tablespoons ground flaxseed and around 6 tablespoons of water, mix and put aside for 15 minutes)

2 tablespoons melted coconut oil

2 tablespoons pure maple syrup

½ cup natural creamy peanut butter

2 ripe bananas

Add-in Ingredients

½ cup finely chopped walnuts

½ cup raisins Optional Topping

2 tablespoons chopped walnuts

2 tablespoons raisins

Directions:

Preheat the oven to 325 degrees F, and then use parchment paper to line a baking sheet and put aside. Add the bananas in a large bowl, and then use a fork to mash them until smooth. Add in the other wet Ingredients and mix until well incorporated. Add the dry Ingredients and then use a rubber spatula to stir and fold them into the dry Ingredients until well mixed. Stir in the walnuts and raisins. Scoop the cookie dough onto the prepared baking sheet making sure that you leave adequate space between the cookies. Bake in the preheated oven for around 12 minutes. Once ready, let the cookies cool on the baking sheet for around 10 minutes. Lift the cookies carefully from the baking sheet onto a cooling rack to further cool. Store the cookies in an airtight container in the fridge or at room temperature for up to one week.

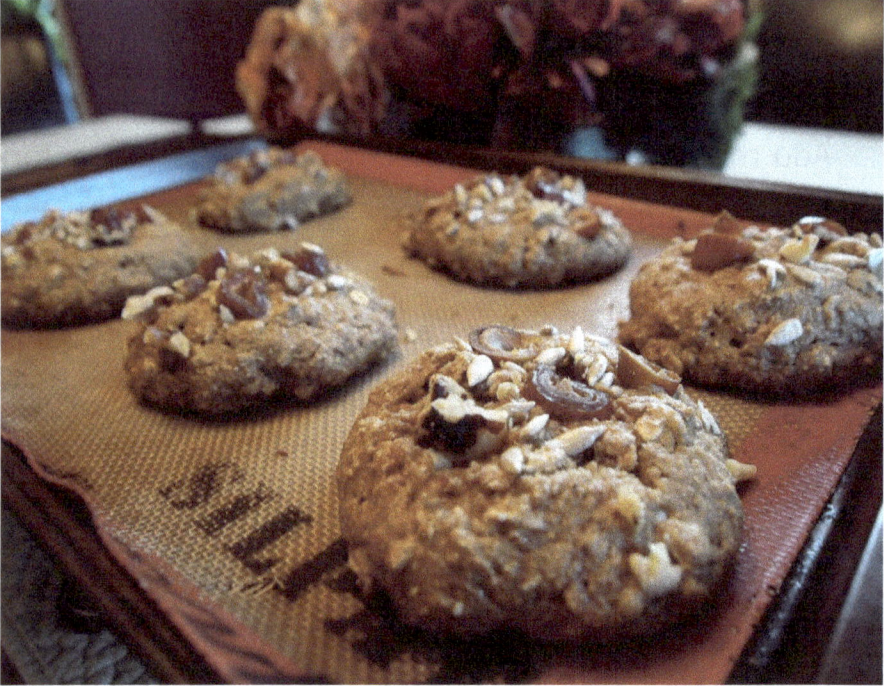

Maca Caramel Frap

Preparation time: 5 minutes

Cooking time: 0 minute

Servings: 4

Ingredients:

1/2 of frozen banana, sliced

1/4 cup cashews, soaked for 4 hours

2 Medjool dates, pitted

1 teaspoon maca powder

1/8 teaspoon sea salt

1/2 teaspoon vanilla extract, unsweetened

1/4 cup almond milk, unsweetened

1/4 cup cold coffee, brewed

Directions:

Place all the ingredients in the order in a food processor or blender and then pulse for 2 to 3 minutes at high speed until smooth. Pour the smoothie into a glass and then serve.

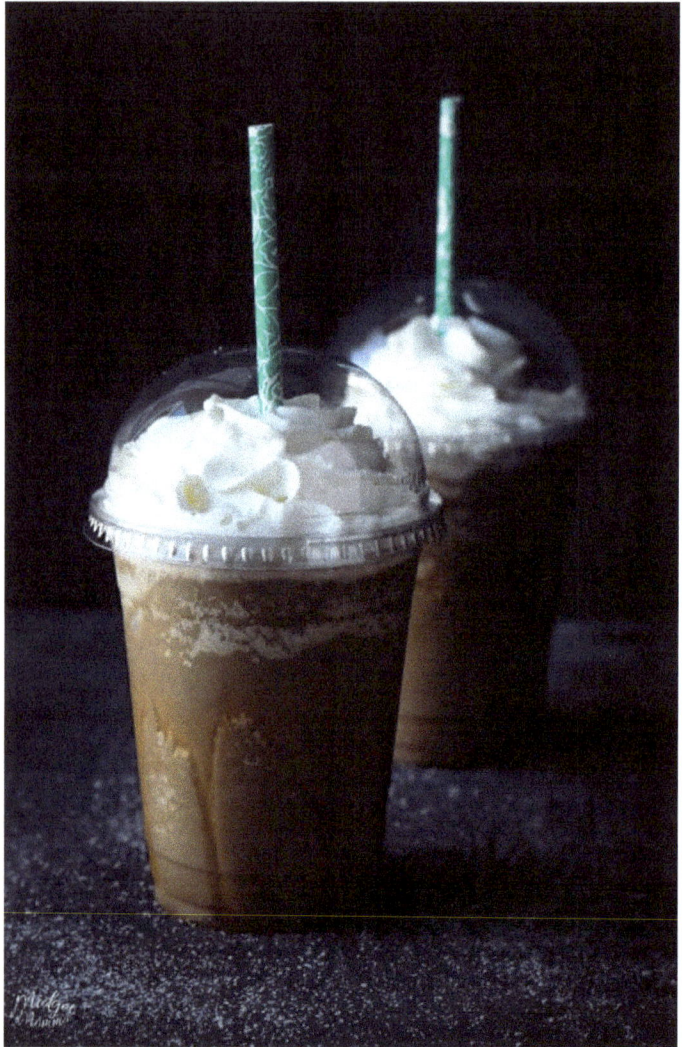

Green Colada

Preparation time: 5 minutes

Cooking time: 0 minute

Servings: 1

Ingredients:

1/2 cup frozen pineapple chunks

1/2 banana

1/2 teaspoon spirulina powder

1/4 teaspoon vanilla extract, unsweetened

1 cup of coconut milk

Directions:

Place all the ingredients in the order in a food processor or blender and then pulse for 2 to 3 minutes at high speed until smooth. Pour the smoothie into a glass and then serve.

Peach Crumble Shake

Preparation time: 5 minutes

Cooking time: 0 minute

Servings: 1

Ingredients:

1 tablespoon chia seeds

¼ cup rolled oats

2 peaches, pitted, sliced

¾ teaspoon ground cinnamon

1 Medjool date, pitted

½ teaspoon vanilla extract, unsweetened

2 tablespoons lemon juice

½ cup of water

1 tablespoon coconut butter

1 cup coconut milk, unsweetened

Directions:

Place all the ingredients in the order in a food processor or blender and then pulse for 2 to 3 minutes at high speed until smooth. Pour the smoothie into a glass and then serve.

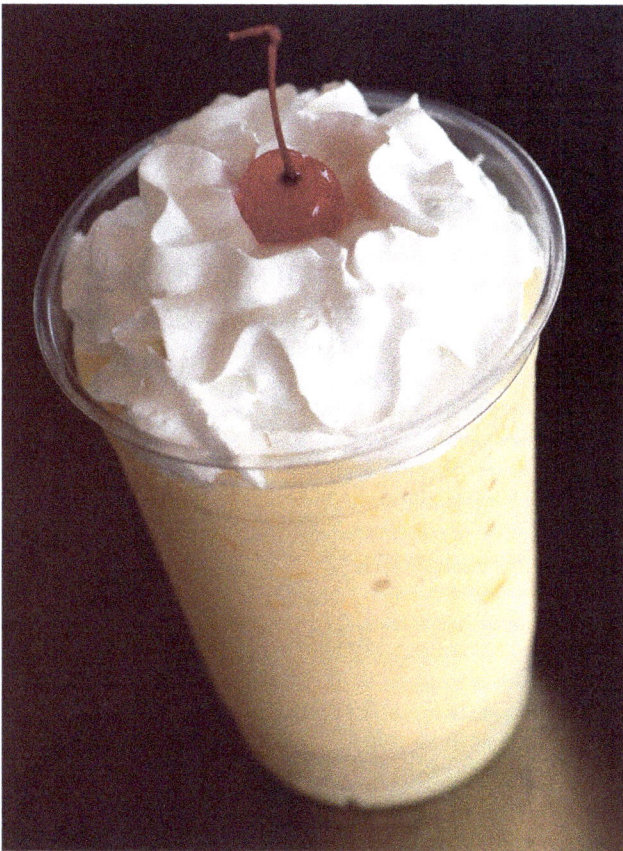

Berry Beet Velvet Smoothie

Preparation time: 5 minutes

Cooking time: 0 minute

Servings: 1

Ingredients:

1/2 of frozen banana

1 cup mixed red berries

1 Medjool date, pitted

1 small beet, peeled, chopped

1 tablespoon cacao powder

1 teaspoon chia seeds

1/4 teaspoon vanilla extract, unsweetened

1/2 teaspoon lemon juice

2 teaspoons coconut butter

1 cup coconut milk, unsweetened

Directions:

Place all the ingredients in the order in a food processor or blender and then pulse for 2 to 3 minutes at high speed until smooth. Pour the smoothie into a glass and then serve.

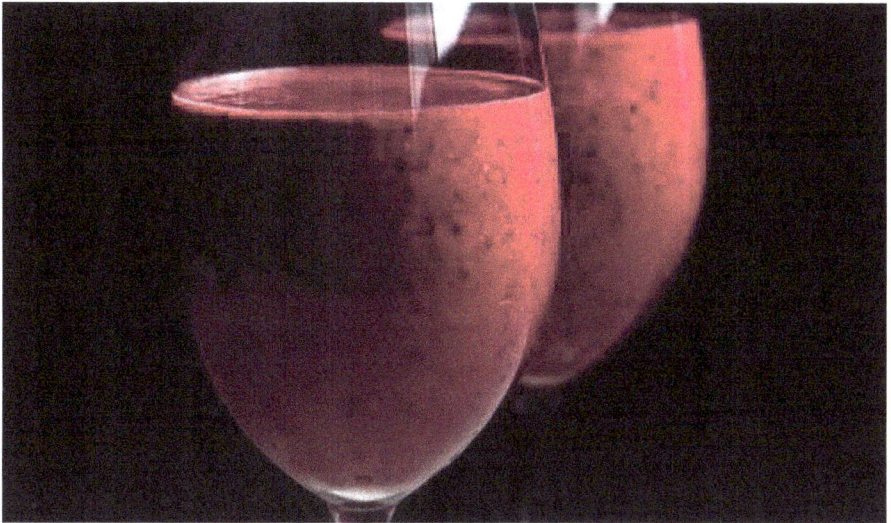

Banana Bread Shake With Walnut Milk

Preparation time: 5 minutes Cooking time: 0 minute
Servings: 2

Ingredients:

2 cups sliced frozen bananas

3 cups walnut milk

1/8 teaspoon grated nutmeg

1 tablespoon maple syrup

1 teaspoon ground cinnamon

1/2 teaspoon vanilla extract, unsweetened

2 tablespoons cacao nibs

Directions:

Place all the ingredients in the order in a food processor or blender and then pulse for 2 to 3 minutes at high speed until smooth. Pour the smoothie into two glasses and then serve.

Strawberry, Banana and Coconut Shake

Preparation time: 5 minutes Cooking time: 0 minute

Servings: 1

Ingredients:

1 tablespoon coconut flakes

1 1/2 cups frozen banana slices

8 strawberries, sliced

1/2 cup coconut milk, unsweetened

1/4 cup strawberries for topping

Directions:

Place all the ingredients in the order in a food processor or blender, except for topping and then pulse for 2 to 3 minutes at high speed until smooth. Pour the smoothie into a glass and then serve.

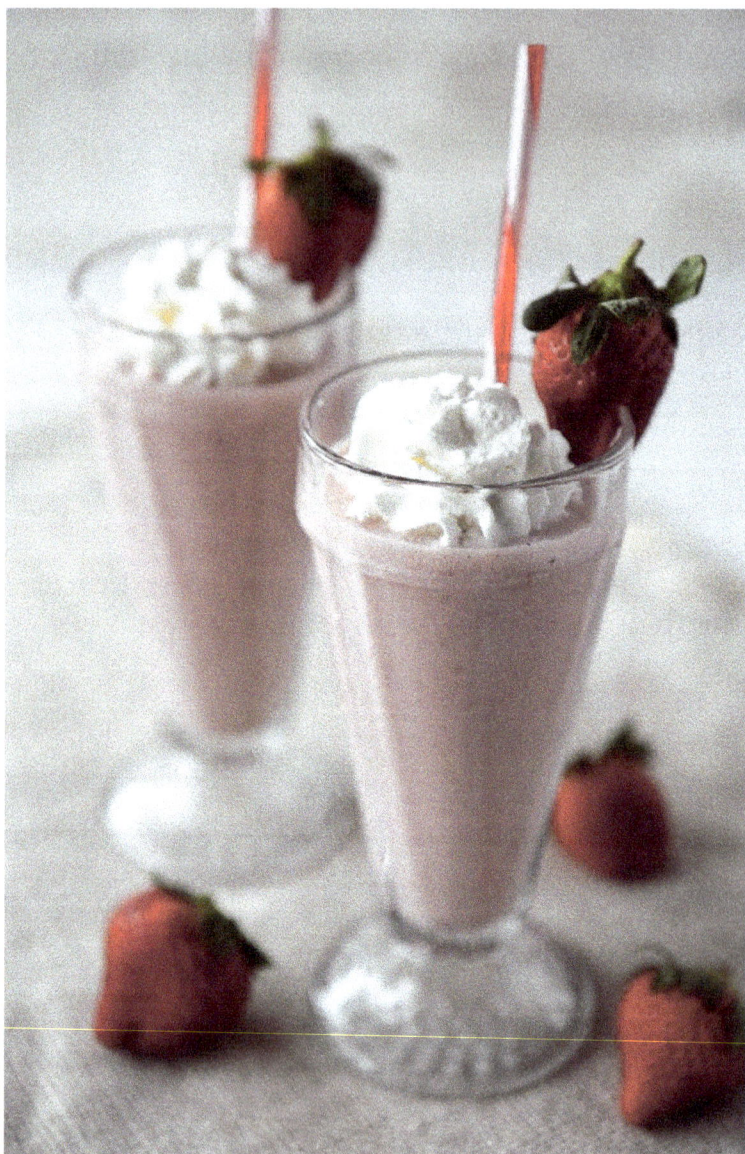

Peanut Butter and Mocha Smoothie

Preparation time: 5 minutes Cooking time: 0 minute Servings: 1

Ingredients:

1 frozen banana, chopped

1 scoop of chocolate protein powder

2 tablespoons rolled oats

1/8 teaspoon sea salt

¼ teaspoon vanilla extract, unsweetened

1 teaspoon cocoa powder, unsweetened

2 tablespoons peanut butter

1 shot of espresso

½ cup almond milk, unsweetened

Directions:

Place all the ingredients in the order in a food processor or blender and then pulse for 2 to 3 minutes at high speed until smooth. Pour the smoothie into a glass and then serve.

Ginger and Greens Smoothie

Preparation time: 5 minutes Cooking time: 0 minute Servings: 1

Ingredients:

1 frozen banana 2 cups baby spinach 2-inch piece of ginger, peeled, chopped ¼ teaspoon cinnamon ¼ teaspoon vanilla extract, unsweetened 1/8 teaspoon salt

1 scoop vanilla protein powder 1/8 teaspoon cayenne pepper 2 tablespoons lemon juice 1 cup of orange juice

Directions:

Place all the ingredients in the order in a food processor or blender and then pulse for 2 to 3 minutes at high speed until smooth. Pour the smoothie into a glass and then serve.

Sweet Potato Smoothie

Preparation time: 5 minutes Cooking time: 0 minute Servings: 1

Ingredients:

1/2 cup frozen zucchini pieces

1 cup cubed cooked sweet potato, frozen

1/2 frozen banana

1/2 teaspoon sea salt

1/2 teaspoon cinnamon

1 scoop of vanilla protein powder

1/4 teaspoon nutmeg

1 tablespoon almond butter

1 1/2 cups almond milk, unsweetened

Directions:

Place all the ingredients in the order in a food processor or blender and then pulse for 2 to 3 minutes at high speed until smooth. Pour the smoothie into a glass and then serve.

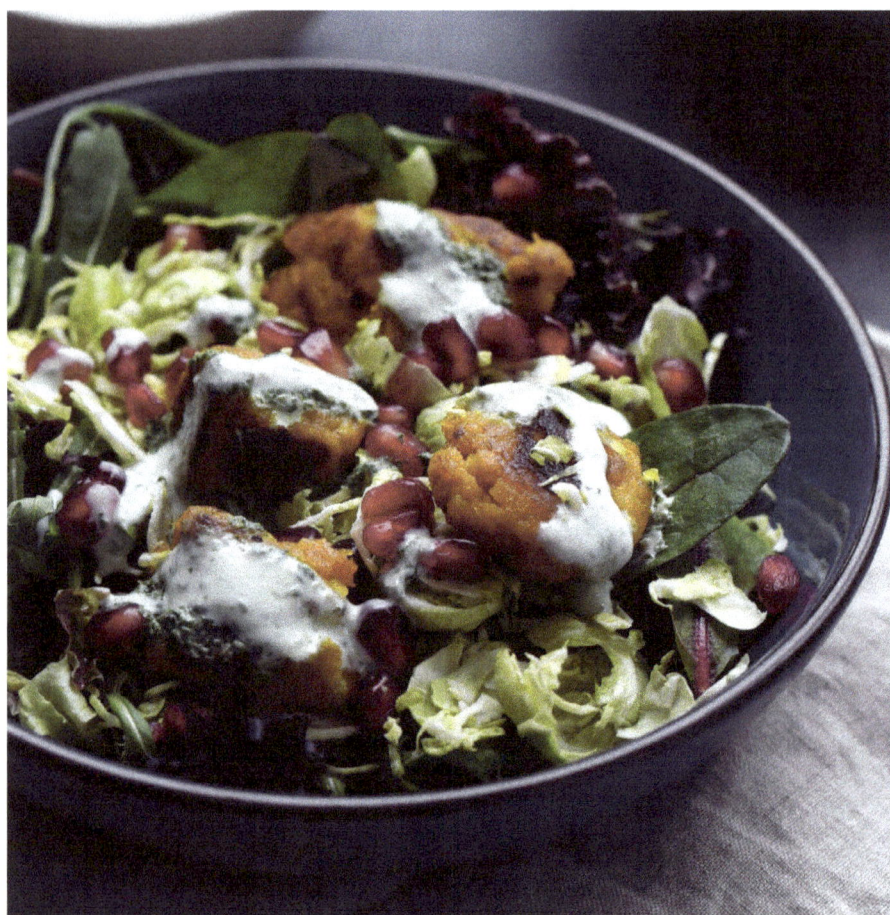

Chocolate Cherry Smoothie

Preparation time: 5 minutes Cooking time: 0 minute
Servings: 1

Ingredients:

1 1/2 cups frozen cherries, pitted

1 cup spinach

1/2 small frozen banana

2 tablespoon cacao powder, unsweetened

1 tablespoon chia seeds

1 scoop of vanilla protein powder

1 teaspoon spirulina

1 1/2 cups almond milk, unsweetened

Directions:

Place all the ingredients in the order in a food processor or blender and then pulse for 2 to 3 minutes at high speed until smooth. Pour the smoothie into a glass and then serve.

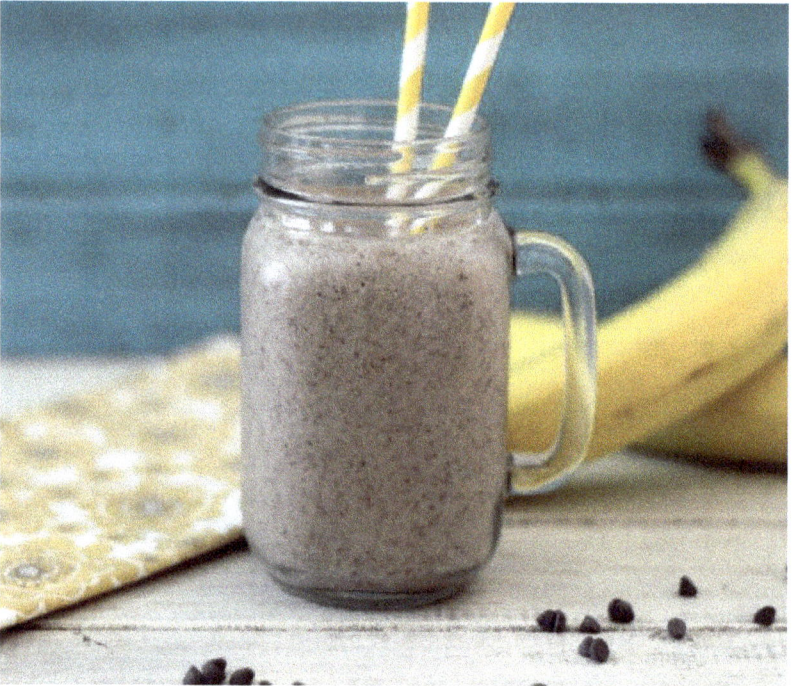

Lemon and Blueberry Smoothie

Preparation time: 5 minutes Cooking time: 0 minute Servings: 1

Ingredients:

1 1/2 cups frozen blueberries

1/2 frozen banana

1 tablespoon chia seeds

3 tablespoon lemon juice

1 teaspoon lemon zest

1 1/2 teaspoon cinnamon

1 1/2 cups almond milk, unsweetened

1 scoop of vanilla protein powder

Directions:

Place all the ingredients in the order in a food processor or blender and then pulse for 2 to 3 minutes at high speed until smooth. Pour the smoothie into a glass and then serve.

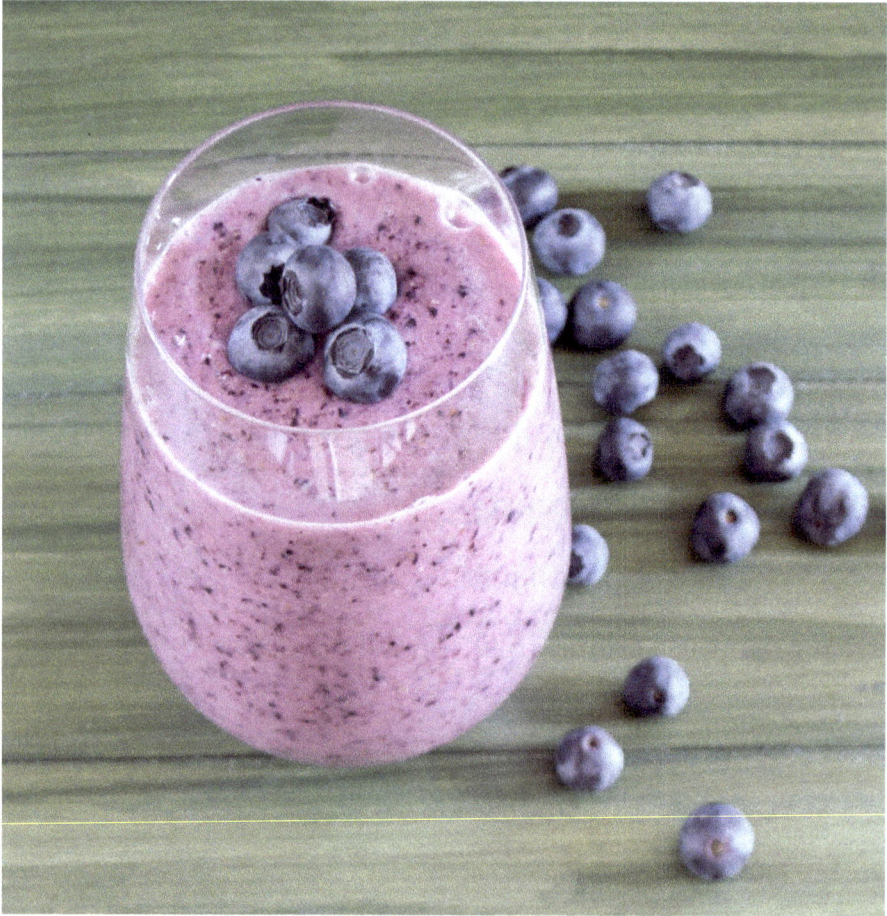

Kale and Spinach Smoothie

Preparation time: 5 minutes Cooking time: 0 minute Servings: 1

Ingredients:

1 cup spinach

1 cup kale

1 frozen banana

3 small dates, pitted

1 1/4 cup almond milk, unsweetened

1 scoop of vanilla protein powder

1 teaspoon cinnamon

Directions:

Place all the ingredients in the order in a food processor or blender and then pulse for 2 to 3 minutes at high speed until smooth. Pour the smoothie into a glass and then serve.

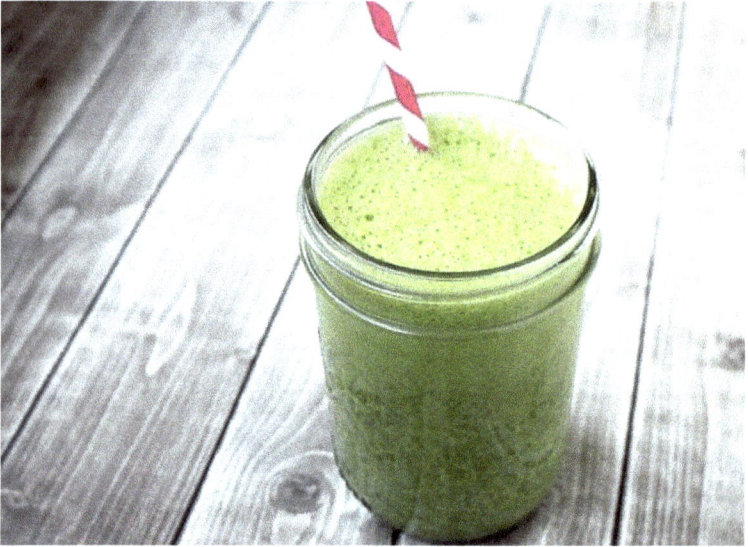

Beet and Orange Smoothie

Preparation time: 5 minutes Cooking time: 0 minute Servings: 1

Ingredients:

1 cup chopped zucchini rounds, frozen

1 cup spinach

1 small peeled navel orange, frozen

1 small chopped beet

1 scoop of vanilla protein powder

1 cup almond milk, unsweetened

Directions:

Place all the ingredients in the order in a food processor or blender and then pulse for 2 to 3 minutes at high speed until smooth. Pour the smoothie into a glass and then serve.

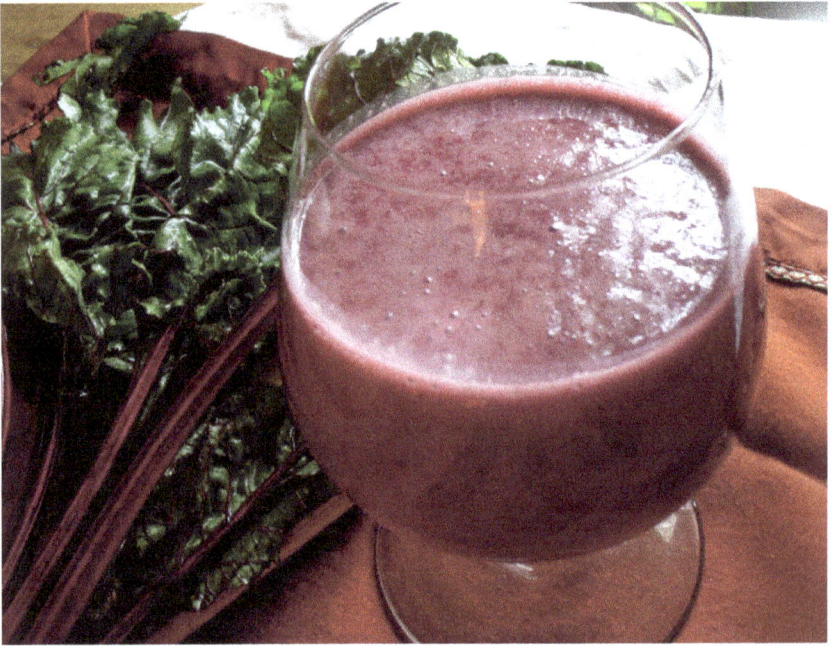

Peanut Butter and Coffee Smoothie

Preparation time: 5 minutes Cooking time: 0 minute
Servings: 1

Ingredients:

2 small frozen banana

1/2 teaspoon ground turmeric

1 tablespoon chia seeds

1 scoop of chocolate protein powder

2 tablespoons Peanut Butter

1 cup strong coffee, brewed

Directions:

Place all the ingredients in the order in a food processor or blender and then pulse for 2 to 3 minutes at high speed until smooth. Pour the smoothie into a glass and then serve.

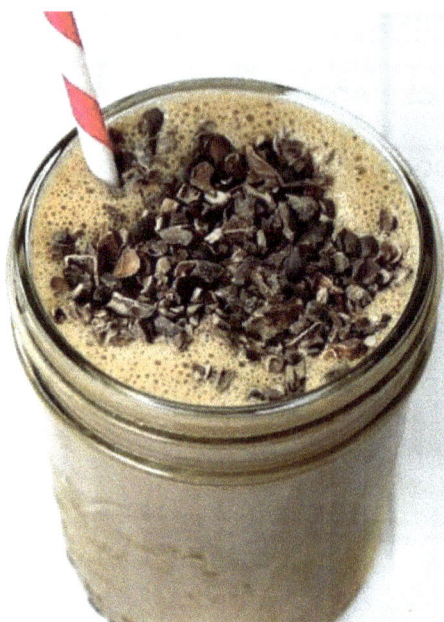

Chocolate, Avocado, and Banana Smoothie

Preparation time: 5 minutes Cooking time: 0 minute Servings: 1

Ingredients:

1 medium frozen banana

2 small dates, pitted

1/2 cup steamed and frozen cauliflower florets

1/4 of a medium avocado

1 teaspoon cinnamon

1 tablespoon cacao powder

1/2 teaspoon sea salt

1 teaspoon maca

1/2 scoop of vanilla protein powder

2 tablespoon cacao nibs

1 tablespoon almond butter

1 cup almond milk

Directions:

Place all the ingredients in the order in a food processor or blender and then pulse for 2 to 3 minutes at high speed until smooth. Pour the smoothie into a glass and then serve.

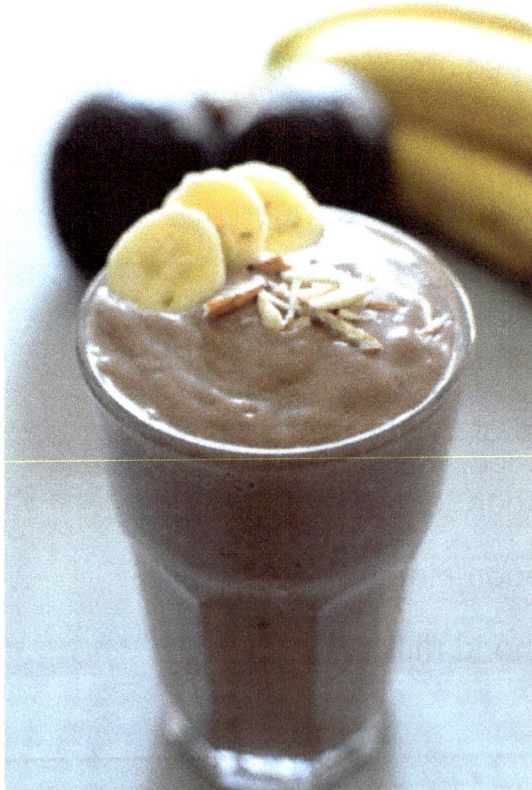

Broccoli and Quinoa Breakfast Patties

Preparation time: 5 minutes Cooking time: 6 minutes
Servings: 4

Ingredients:

1 cup cooked quinoa, cooked

1/2 cup shredded broccoli florets

1/2 cup shredded carrots

2 cloves of garlic, minced

2 teaspoon parsley

1 1/2 teaspoon onion powder

1 1/2 teaspoon garlic powder

1/3 teaspoon salt

1/4 teaspoon black pepper

1/2 cup bread crumbs, gluten-free

2 tablespoon coconut oil 2 flax eggs

Directions:

Prepare patties and for this, place all the ingredients in a large bowl, except for oil and stir until well combined and then shape the mixture into patties. Take a skillet pan, place it over medium heat, add oil and when hot, add prepared patties in it and cook for 3 minutes per side until golden brown and crispy. Serve patties with vegan sour creams.

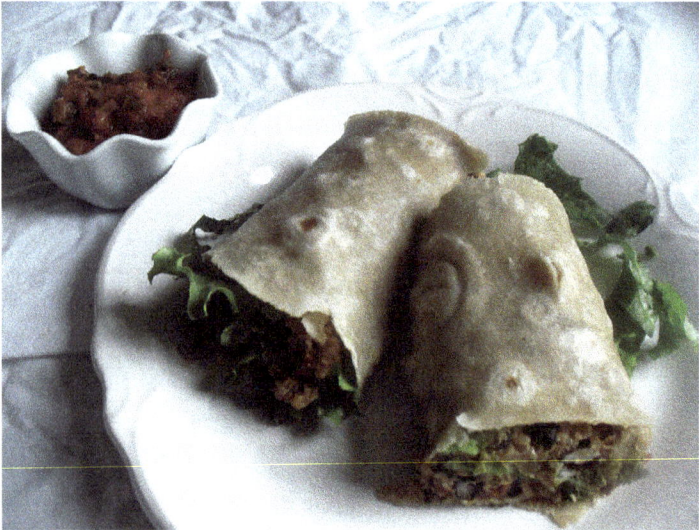

Scrambled Tofu Breakfast Tacos

Preparation time: 5 minutes Cooking time: 10 minutes
Servings: 4

Ingredients:

12 ounces tofu, pressed, drained

1/2 cup grape tomatoes, quartered

1 medium red pepper, diced

1 medium avocado, sliced

1 clove of garlic, minced

1/4 teaspoon ground turmeric

1/4 teaspoon ground black pepper

1/4 teaspoon salt

1/4 teaspoon cumin

1 teaspoon olive oil

8 corn tortillas

Directions:

Take a skillet pan, place it over medium heat, add oil and when hot, add pepper and garlic and cook for 2 minutes. Then add tofu, crumble it, sprinkle with black pepper, salt, and all the spices, stir and cook for 5 minutes. When done, distribute tofu between tortilla, top with tomato and avocado, and serve.

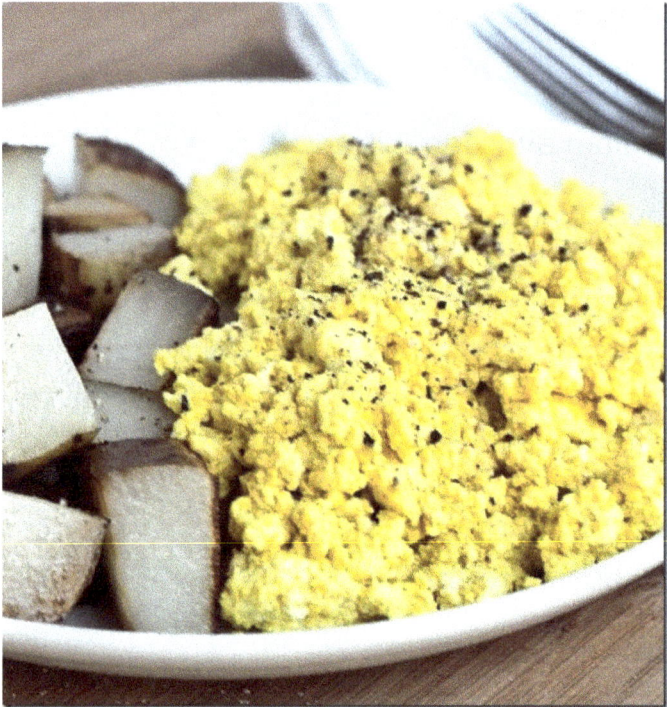

Sweet Potato Breakfast Hash

Preparation time: 5 minutes Cooking time: 28 minutes
Servings: 4

Ingredients:

4 cups cubed sweet potatoes, peeled

1/2 teaspoon sea salt

1/2 teaspoon turmeric

1/2 teaspoon cumin

1 teaspoon smoked paprika

2 cups diced white onion

2 cloves of garlic, peeled, minced

1/4 cup chopped cilantro

1 tablespoon coconut oil

½ cup vegan guacamole, for serving

1 ½ cup pica de Gallo

Directions:

Take a skillet pan, place it over medium heat, add oil and
when it melts, add onion, potatoes, and garlic, season

with salt, paprika, turmeric, and cumin, stir and cook for 25 minutes until potatoes are slightly caramelized. Then remove the pan from heat, add cilantro and distribute evenly between serving plates. Top the sweet potato hash with guacamole and pico de gallo and then serve.

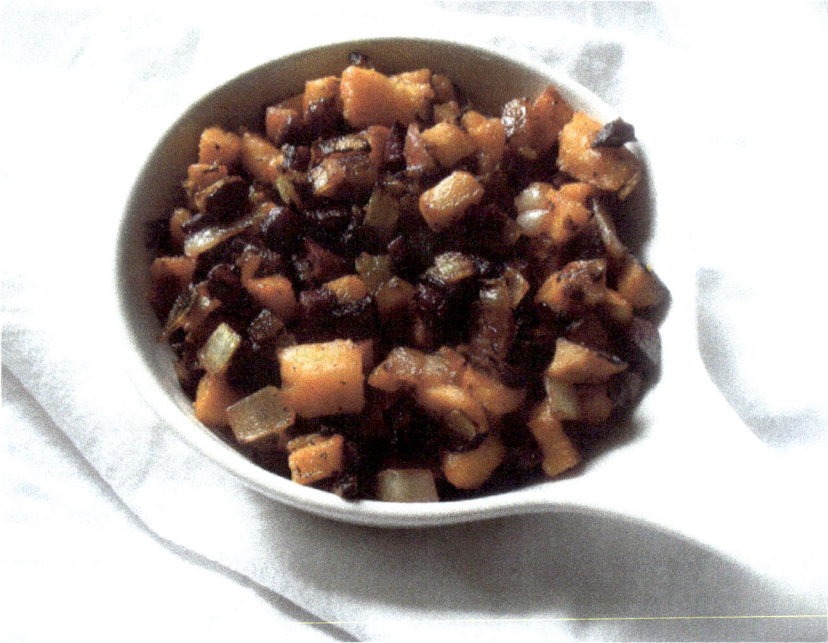

Chocolate Chip, Strawberry and Oat Waffles

Preparation time: 10 minutes Cooking time: 25 minutes

Servings: 6

Ingredients:

6 tablespoons chocolate chips, semi-sweet

½ cup chopped strawberries

Powdered sugar as needed for topping

Dry 1/4 cup oats

1 1/2 tablespoon ground flaxseeds

1 1/2 cup whole wheat pastry flour

2 1/2 tablespoon cocoa powder

1/4 teaspoon salt

2 teaspoons baking powder

Wet Ingredients:

1/3 cup mashed bananas

2 tablespoon maple syrup

2 tablespoon coconut oil

1/2 teaspoon vanilla extract, unsweetened

1/4 cup applesauce, unsweetened

1 3/4 cup almond milk, unsweetened

Directions:

Take a medium bowl, place all the dry ingredients in it, and whisk until mixed. Take a large bowl, place all the wet ingredients in it, whisk until combined, and then whisk in dry ingredients mixture in four batches until incorporated, don't overmix. Let the batter stand at room temperature for 5 minutes and in the meantime, switch on the waffle iron and let it preheat until hot. Then ladle one-sixth of the batter in it and cook until golden brown and firm. Cook remaining waffles in the same manner and when done, top them with chocolate chips and berries, sprinkle with sugar and then serve.

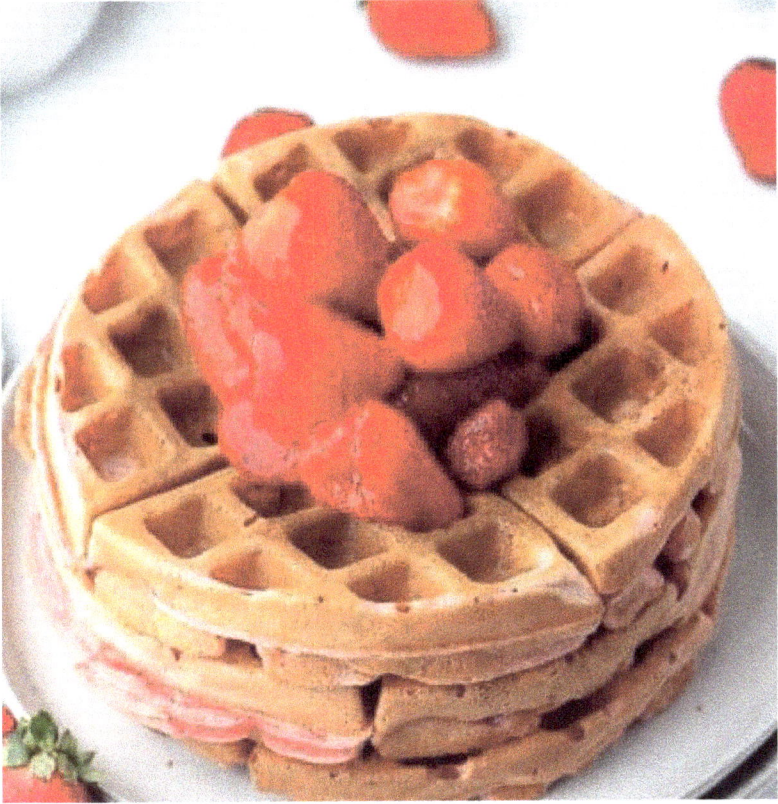

Scrambled Eggs with Aquafaba

Preparation time: 5 minutes Cooking time: 15 minutes Servings: 2

Ingredients:

6 ounces tofu, firm, pressed, drained

1/2 cup aquafaba

1 1/2 tablespoons olive oil

1 tablespoon nutritional yeast

1/4 teaspoon black salt

1/8 teaspoon ground turmeric

1/4 teaspoon ground black pepper

Directions:

Take a food processor, add tofu, yeast, black pepper, salt, and turmeric, then pour in aquafaba and olive oil and pulse for 1 minute until smooth. Take a skillet pan, place it over medium heat, and when hot, add tofu mixture and cook for 1 minute. Cover the pan, continue cooking for 3 minutes, then uncover the pan and pull the mixture across the pan with a wooden spoon until soft forms. Continue cooking for 10 minutes until resembles soft scrambled eggs, folding tofu mixture gently and heat over medium heat, then remove the pan from heat and season with salt and black pepper to taste. Serve straight away.

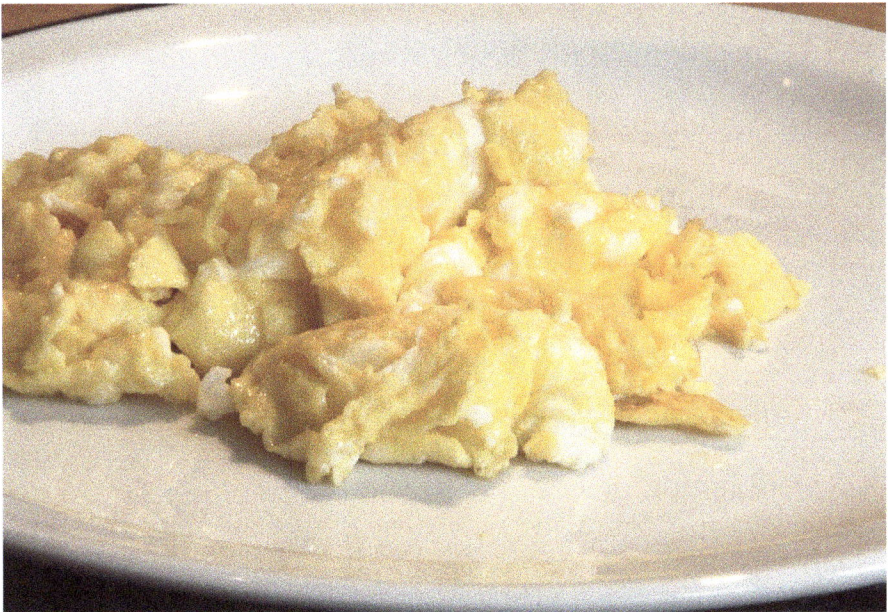

Sweet Potato and Apple Latkes

Preparation time: 5 minutes Cooking time: 15 minutes

Servings: 4

Ingredients:

1 large sweet potato, peeled, grated

1/2 of medium white onion, diced

1 apple, peeled, cored, grated

2 tablespoons spelt flour

1 tablespoon arrowroot powder

½ teaspoon cracked black pepper

1 teaspoon salt

1 teaspoon turmeric

1 tablespoon olive oil and more for frying

Tahini lemon drizzle, for serving

Directions:

Wrap grated potato and apple in a cheesecloth, then squeeze moisture as much as possible and then place in a bowl. Add remaining ingredients and then stir until combined. Take a skillet pan, place it over medium-high heat, add oil and when hot, drop in prepared batter, shape them into a round patty and cook for 4 minutes per side until crispy and brown. Serve latkes with Tahini lemon drizzle.

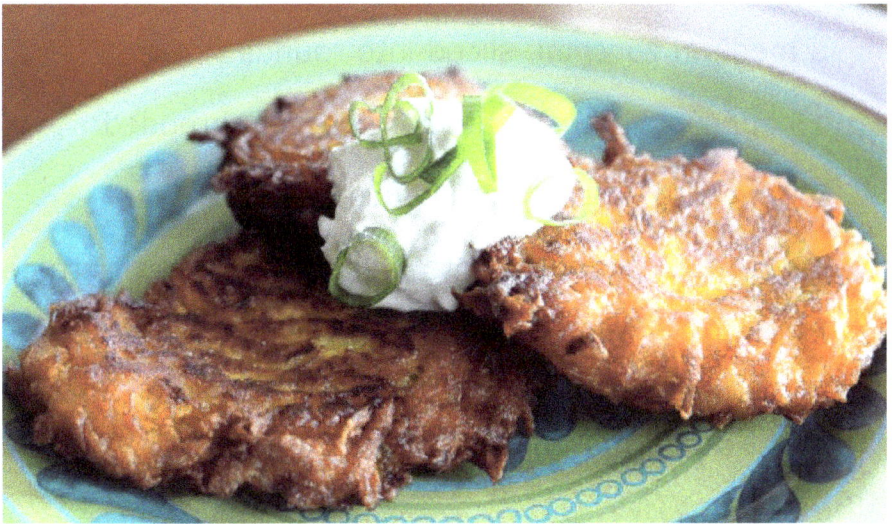

Enchilada Breakfast Casserole

Preparation time: 10 minutes Cooking time: 25 minutes Servings: 8

Ingredients:

15 ounces cooked corn

1 batch of vegan breakfast eggs

15 ounces cooked pinto beans

3 medium zucchini, sliced into rounds

10 ounces of vegan cheddar cheese, shredded

24 ounces red enchilada sauce

12 corn tortillas, cut into wedges Shredded lettuce for serving Vegan sour cream for serving

Directions:

Take a skillet pan, grease it with oil and press the vegan breakfast eggs into the bottom of the pan in an even layer. Spread with 1/3 of enchilada sauce, then sprinkle with half of the cheese and cover with half of the tortilla wedges. Cover the wedges with 1/3 of the sauce, then layer with beans, corn, and zucchini, cover with remaining tortilla wedges, and spread the remaining sauce on top. Cover the pan with lid, place it over medium heat and cook for 25 minutes until cheese had melted, zucchini is tender, and sauce is bubbling. When done, let the casserole stand for 10 minutes, top with lettuce and sour cream, then cut the casserole into wedges, and serve.

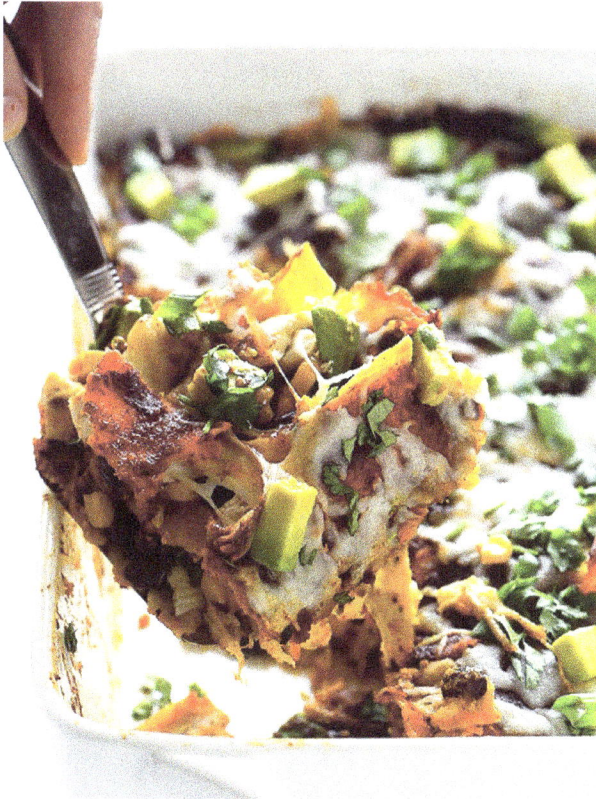

Vegan Breakfast Sandwich

Preparation time: 15 minutes Cooking time: 8 minutes

Servings: 3

Ingredients:

1 cup of spinach

6 slices of pickle

14 oz tofu , extra-firm, pressed

2 medium tomatoes , sliced

1/2 teaspoon garlic powder

¼ teaspoon ground black pepper

1/2 teaspoon black salt

1 teaspoon turmeric

1 tablespoon coconut oil

2 tablespoons vegan mayo

3 slices of vegan cheese

6 slices of gluten-free bread, toasted

Directions:

Cut tofu into six slices, and then season its one side with garlic, black pepper, salt, and turmeric. Take a skillet pan, place it over medium heat, add oil and when hot, add seasoned tofu slices in it, season side down, and cook for 3 minutes until crispy and light brown. Then flip the tofu slices and continue cooking for 3 minutes until browned and crispy. When done, transfer tofu slices on a baking sheet, in the form of a set of two slices side by side, then top each set with a cheese slice and broil for 3 minutes until cheese has melted. Spread mayonnaise on both sides of slices, top with two slices of tofu, cheese on the side, top with spinach, tomatoes, pickles, and then close the sandwich. Cut the sandwich into half and then serve.

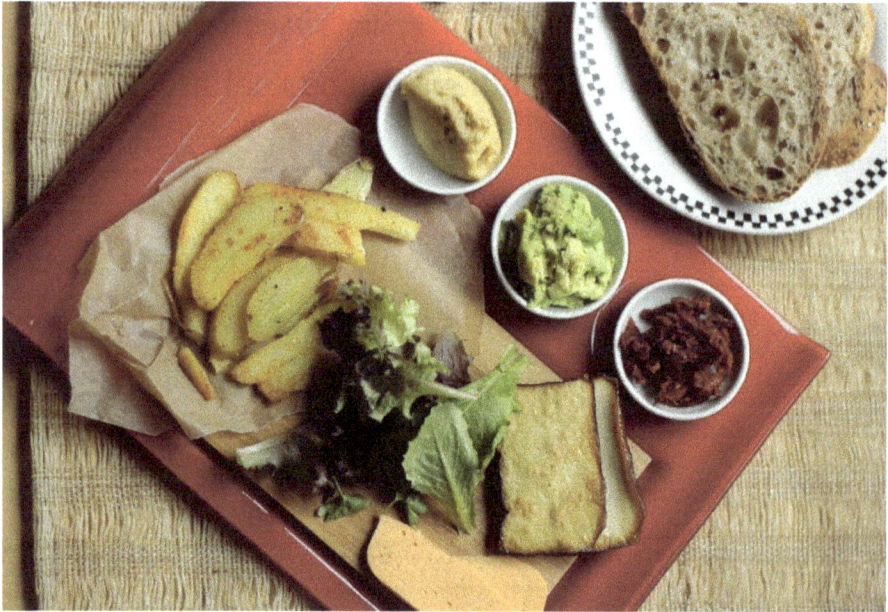

Sweet Crepes

Preparation time: 5 minutes Cooking time: 8 minutes Servings: 5

Ingredients:

1 cup of water

1 banana

1/2 cup oat flour

1/2 cup brown rice flour

1 teaspoon baking powder

1 tablespoon coconut sugar

1/8 teaspoon salt

Directions:

Take a blender, place all the ingredients in it except for sugar and salt and pulse for 1 minute until smooth. Take a skillet pan, place it over medium-high heat, grease it with oil and when hot, pour in ¼ cup of batter, spread it as thin as possible, and cook for 2 to 3 minutes per side until golden brown. Cook remaining crepes in the same manner, then sprinkle with sugar and salt and serve.

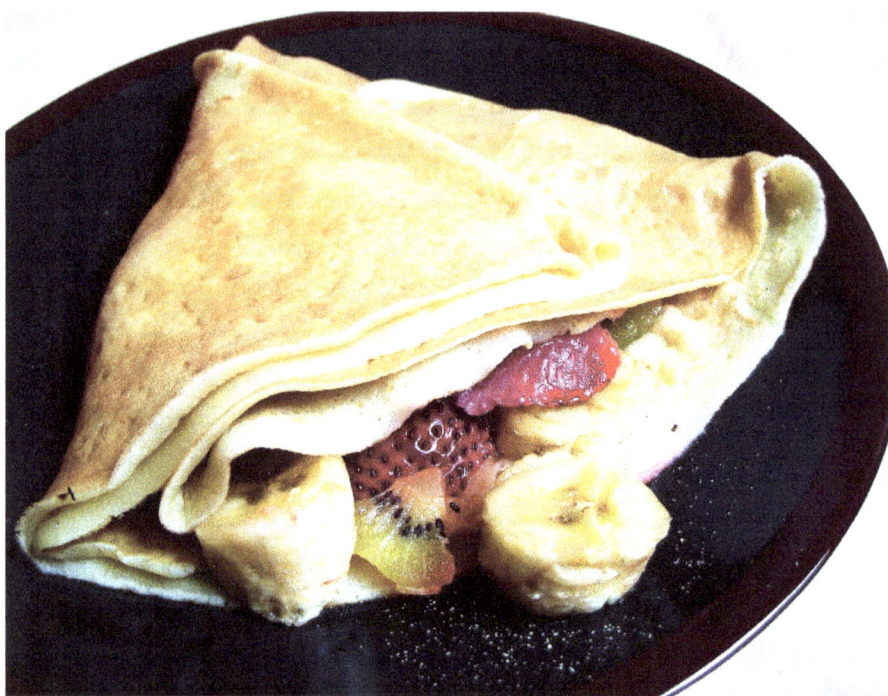

www.ingramcontent.com/pod-product-compliance
Lightning Source LLC
Chambersburg PA
CBHW050752030426
42336CB00012B/1787